MIND DIET COOKBOOK FOR SENIORS OVER 60

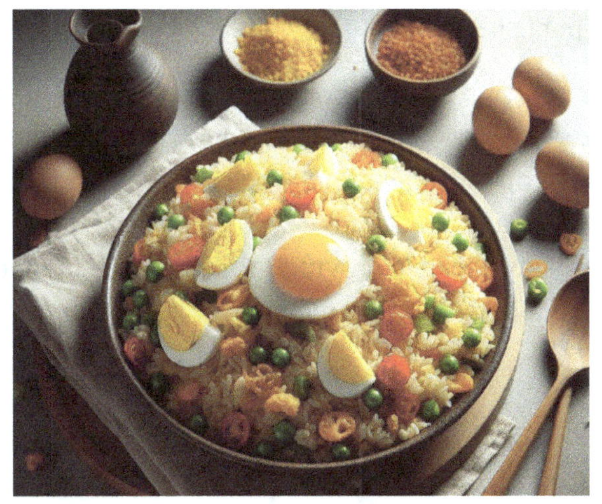

Flavorful Recipes to Boost Brainpower and Prevent Alzheimer's and Dementia

Robert Elliot

Table of Contents

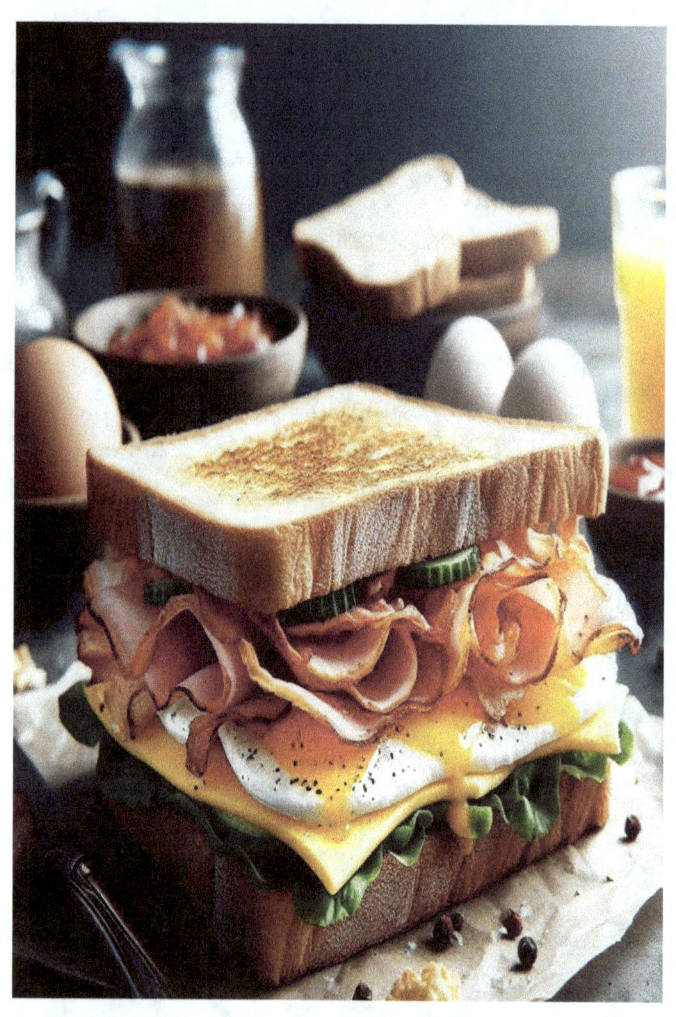

Introduction

When my big aunty, Aunt Jane, started humming show tunes in the checkout line at Walmart, I knew something was up. This was the woman who mastered the silent stare – that laser beam that could melt butter and shrink credit card debt. Now, she was belting out "Don't Rain on My Parade" like Barbra Streisand on a karaoke bender.

Sure, I'm a nutritionist extraordinaire, but even I got thrown when my sassy 64-year-old aunty went full Broadway at checkout aisle 4. Turns out, it wasn't a spontaneous musical awakening. It was the MIND diet. Yes, that one backed by scientific studies with names so long they trip your tongue. Trust me, I was skeptical too. But then I saw the change.

The woman who forgot where she parked her keys – now remembering everyone's birthday. The lady who could barely climb the stairs – walking briskly past me at the park. And those show tunes? Let's just say the neighborhood squirrels learned a whole new repertoire.

This wasn't some magic pill, folks. This was food. Delicious, soul-warming, flavor-packed food that was actually sharpening Aunt Jane's mind like a diamond in a blender. I felt compelled to share it.

Because if it could turn my fiercely independent aunty into a singing, strutting dynamo, imagine what it could do for you.

Forget the crossword puzzles and brain games. Ditch the supplements and pricey powders. This book isn't about trendy fads or quick fixes. It's about fueling your brain with the very stuff that keeps it young – the stuff that makes you sharper, wittier, and yes, maybe even a little bolder.

This is your roadmap to a MIND revolution on your plate. We're talking vibrant salads that punch like Muhammad Ali, berry smoothies that taste like a party in your mouth, and salmon dishes that'll make you rewrite your definition of "comfort food." It's easy to make, tasty, and supported by science that wouldn't lie to its grandmother.

So, crack open this book, grab your apron, and get ready to cook up a storm. Because you're not just feeding your body, you're feeding your future. And who knows? Maybe by the time you finish the last recipe, you'll be belting out your own show tune in the produce aisle. Now, that's worth singing about.

Ready to unlock your MIND's full potential? Let's do this.

Chapter 1: Understanding the MIND Diet

Welcome to the transformative world of the MIND diet—an innovative approach specifically designed to support and enhance cognitive function, especially for seniors aged 60 and beyond. In this chapter, we will delve into the core principles of the MIND diet, unveiling the science behind its creation and exploring the profound connection between nutrition and cognitive health.

The Origins of the MIND Diet

The MIND diet, short for Mediterranean-DASH Intervention for Neurodegenerative Delay, is a fusion of two renowned dietary approaches: the Mediterranean Diet and the DASH (Dietary Approaches to Stop Hypertension) Diet. Developed by researchers, this unique blend has shown promising results in studies, suggesting a correlation between adherence to the MIND diet and a reduced risk of neurodegenerative diseases, including Alzheimer's.

Core Principles of the MIND Diet

Understanding the key principles of the MIND diet is crucial to its successful implementation. This diet emphasizes the consumption of specific nutrients that have been scientifically linked to brain health. Key components include:

- **Leafy Greens**: Packed with antioxidants and essential nutrients, leafy greens like kale and spinach are staples in the MIND diet, promoting cognitive function.

- **Berries**: Blueberries, in particular, have been identified as potent brain-boosting fruits. Their high levels of antioxidants contribute to improved memory and cognitive abilities.

- **Nuts and Seeds**: Rich in omega-3 fatty acids and other beneficial nutrients, nuts and seeds play a vital role in supporting overall brain health.

- **Whole Grains**: Complex carbohydrates found in whole grains provide a steady release of energy, crucial for maintaining focus and concentration.

- **Fish**: Fatty fish, such as salmon and trout, are excellent sources of omega-3 fatty acids, essential for brain structure and function.

- **Olive Oil**: A staple in the Mediterranean Diet, olive oil is a healthy fat that has been associated with cognitive benefits.

The Science of Nutrition and Cognitive Function

Delving into the science behind the MIND diet, we'll explore how specific nutrients impact cognitive function. From antioxidants combating oxidative stress to omega-3 fatty acids supporting brain cell structure, understanding these mechanisms will empower you to make informed and intentional choices when it comes to your diet.

As you embark on this MIND diet journey, remember that the choices you make in your kitchen can have a profound impact on the health and vitality of your brain. Stay tuned as we guide you through practical tips and delicious recipes designed to nourish your mind and promote longevity.

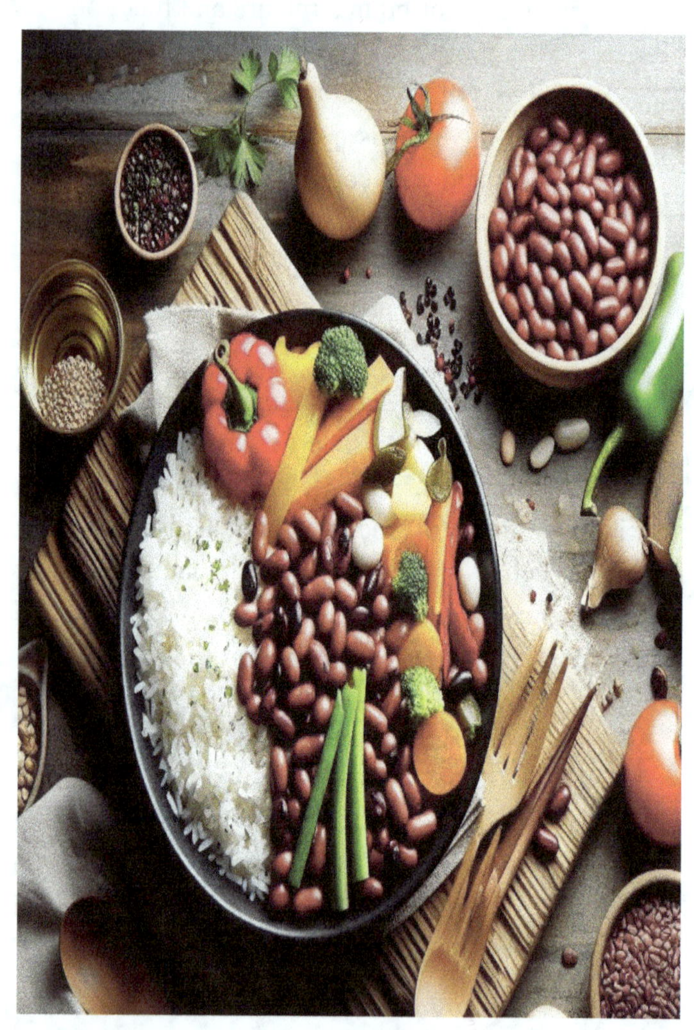

Chapter 2: Stocking Your Kitchen

Now that we've uncovered the foundational principles of the MIND diet, it's time to set the stage for success by stocking your kitchen with brain-boosting essentials. In this chapter, we'll explore the key ingredients that will become the building blocks of your cognitive well-being, as well as offer practical tips for mindful grocery shopping.

Essential Ingredients for Brain-Boosting Meals

1. Leafy Greens

Ensure your refrigerator is stocked with an array of nutrient-dense leafy greens such as kale, spinach, and Swiss chard. These powerhouses of vitamins, minerals, and antioxidants form the backbone of MIND diet meals.

2. Berries

Keep a variety of berries on hand, including blueberries, strawberries, and raspberries. Their rich colors signify high levels of brain-friendly antioxidants that contribute to cognitive health.

3. Nuts and Seeds

Create a convenient snack station with a mix of nuts and seeds like walnuts, almonds, chia seeds, and flaxseeds. These provide essential omega-3 fatty acids and other nutrients crucial for brain function.

4. Whole Grains

Opt for whole grains such as brown rice, quinoa, and oats. These complex carbohydrates release energy steadily, supporting sustained focus and mental clarity throughout the day.

5. Fatty Fish

Include a variety of fatty fish in your freezer, such as salmon, mackerel, and sardines. These are rich in omega-3 fatty acids, promoting optimal brain health.

6. Olive Oil

It is very important that you choose extra virgin olive oil as your go-to cooking oil. Its monounsaturated fats and antioxidants make it a key component of the MIND diet.

Tips for Mindful Grocery Shopping

1. Make a List and Stick to It

Make a thorough shopping list and plan your meals for the next week before you go to the grocery store. This ensures you stay focused on purchasing the essential MIND diet ingredients.

2. Shop the Perimeter

In most grocery stores, fresh produce, lean proteins, and whole grains are typically located around the perimeter. Concentrate your shopping in these areas to fill your cart with brain-boosting options.

3. Choose Colorful Produce

Vibrant, colorful fruits and vegetables often contain a variety of beneficial compounds. Aim for a rainbow on your plate to maximize the nutritional diversity of your meals.

4. Read Labels Mindfully

When selecting packaged foods, pay attention to nutritional labels. Opt for items with minimal processing and low added sugars, keeping in line with the MIND diet's emphasis on whole, natural foods.

Armed with a well-stocked kitchen and mindful shopping habits, you're ready to embark on a MINDful cooking journey. The next chapters will guide you through delicious and brain-nourishing recipes to make the most of these nutritious ingredients.

Chapter 3: Breakfast Recipes

Shrimp And Eggs Mix

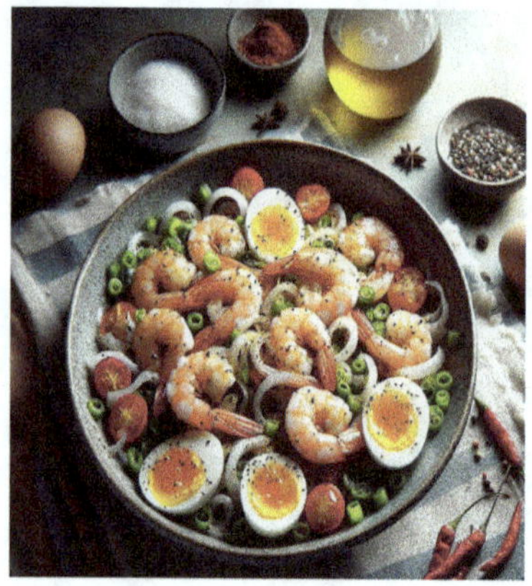

Preparation Time: 15 minutes
Cooking Time: 10 minutes
Servings: 2

Ingredients:
- 200g shrimp, peeled and deveined
- 4 eggs
- Salt and pepper to taste
- 2 tbsp olive oil
- Fresh herbs for garnish

Directions:

1. In a nonstick pan, heat up one tablespoon of olive oil over medium heat.

2. Add peeled and deveined shrimp to the pan, season with salt and pepper, and cook until they turn pink and opaque, about 3-4 minutes. Remove the shrimp from the pan and set aside.

3. Add one more tablespoon of olive oil to the same pan.

4. Crack the eggs into a bowl, whisk, and pour them into the pan.

5. Scramble the eggs until fully cooked, then add the cooked shrimp back to the pan and mix well.

6. Garnish with fresh herbs and serve hot.

Nutritional Values (per serving):
Calories: 300 | Fat: 20g | Protein: 25g |
Carbs: 2g | Fiber: 0.5g | Sugar: 0.5g |
Sodium: 400mg

Savory Breakfast Sandwich

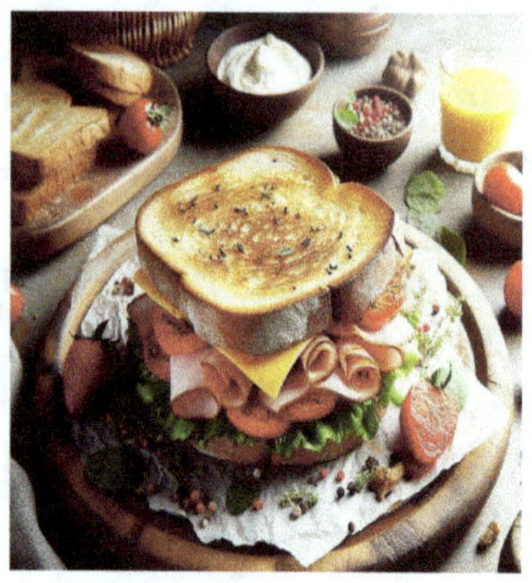

Preparation Time: 10 minutes
Cooking Time: 5 minutes
Servings: 1

Ingredients:
- 1 whole-grain English muffin
- 1 egg
- 1 slice of turkey or chicken
- 1 slice of cheese
- Spinach leaves

Directions:
1. Toast the whole-grain English muffin.
2. In a skillet, cook the egg to your liking (fried or scrambled).
3. Assemble the sandwich by placing the cooked egg on the bottom half of the English muffin.

4. Add a slice of turkey or chicken, a slice of cheese, and fresh spinach leaves.

5. Top with the other half of the English muffin and press gently.

Nutritional Values (per serving):
Calories: 350 | Fat: 15g | Protein: 20g |
Carbs: 30g | Fiber: 5g | Sugar: 3g |
Sodium: 450mg

Almond Quinoa

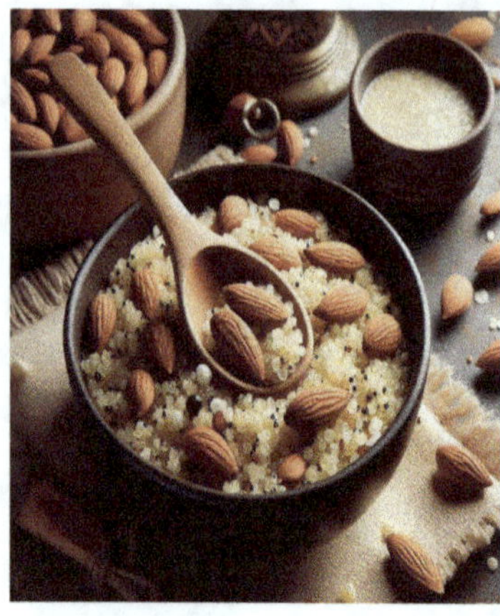

Preparation Time: 20 minutes
Cooking Time: 15 minutes
Servings: 4

Ingredients:
- 1 cup quinoa
- 2 cups almond milk
- 1/2 cup almonds, chopped
- 1 tbsp honey
- Fresh berries for topping

Directions:
1. Rinse 1 cup of quinoa under cold water.
2. In a saucepan, combine quinoa and 2 cups of almond milk. Bring to a boil.
3. Reduce heat, cover, and simmer for 15 minutes or until quinoa is cooked and liquid is absorbed.

4. In a separate pan, toast the chopped almonds until golden brown.

5. Once quinoa is cooked, stir in the toasted almonds and honey.

6. Serve in bowls, topped with fresh berries.

Nutritional Values (per serving):
Calories: 280 | Fat: 12g | Protein: 8g |
Carbs: 35g | Fiber: 5g | Sugar: 8g |
Sodium: 200mg

Coconut Buckwheat Porridge

Prep Time: 10 minutes | Cooking Time: 15 minutes | Servings: 3

Ingredients:
- 1 cup buckwheat groats
- 2 cups coconut milk
- 1/4 cup shredded coconut
- 1 banana, sliced
- Maple syrup for drizzling

Directions:
1. Rinse 1 cup of buckwheat groats under cold water.
2. In a saucepan, combine buckwheat groats and 2 cups of coconut milk. Bring to a simmer.
3. Cook for 15 minutes or until the buckwheat is tender and the liquid is absorbed.
4. Stir in shredded coconut.
5. Serve in bowls, topped with banana slices and a drizzle of maple syrup.

Nutritional Values (per serving):
Calories: 320 | Fat: 15g | Protein: 9g |
Carbs: 40g | Fiber: 6g | Sugar: 10g |
Sodium: 100mg

Scrambled Tofu

Prep Time: 15 minutes | Cooking Time: 10 minutes | Servings: 3

Ingredients:
- 1 block of firm tofu, crumbled
- 1 tbsp olive oil
- 1/2 onion, diced
- 1 bell pepper, diced
- 1 tsp turmeric
- Salt and pepper to taste

Directions:
1. In a skillet set over medium heat, preheat 1 tablespoon of olive oil.
2. Sauté diced onion and bell pepper until softened.
3. Add the crumbled tofu to the skillet, sprinkle turmeric, salt, and pepper.
4. Cook, stirring occasionally, until the tofu is heated through and slightly golden.
5. Adjust seasoning as needed and serve hot.

Nutritional Values (per serving):
Calories: 180 | Fat: 10g | Protein: 15g |
Carbs: 10g | Fiber: 3g | Sugar: 2g |
Sodium: 300mg

Spinach Omelet

Prep Time: 10 minutes | Cooking Time: 5 minutes | Servings: 1

Ingredients:
- 2 eggs
- Handful of fresh spinach
- 1/4 cup feta cheese, crumbled
- Salt and pepper to taste

Directions:
1. Crack 2 eggs into a bowl, whisk, and season with salt and pepper.
2. Heat a non-stick skillet over medium heat.
3. Pour the whisked eggs into the skillet, covering the bottom evenly.
4. Add fresh spinach and crumbled feta on one half of the eggs.
5. Once the eggs start to set, fold the other half over the spinach and feta.
6. Cook until the eggs are fully set and the cheese is melted.

Nutritional Values (per serving):
Calories: 250 | Fat: 18g | Protein: 18g |
Carbs: 4g | Fiber: 2g | Sugar: 1g |
Sodium: 400mg

Belgian Waffles

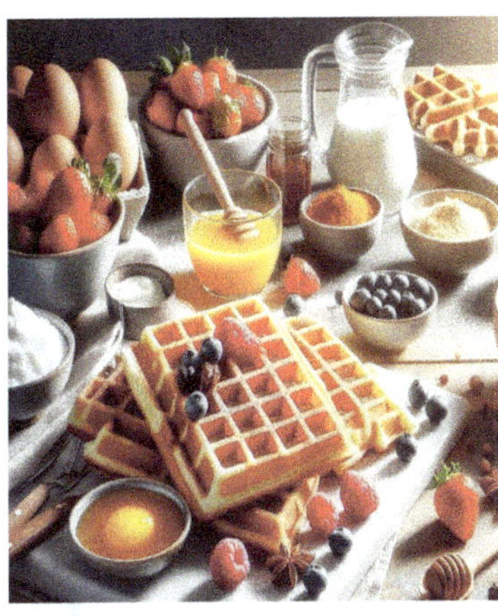

Preparation Time: 20 minutes
Cooking Time: 5 minutes each
Servings: 4

Ingredients:
- 2 cups flour
- 1 tbsp sugar
- 2 tsp baking powder
- 1/2 tsp salt
- 1 3/4 cups milk
- 1/3 cup vegetable oil
- 2 eggs

Directions:
1. Mix the flour, sugar, baking powder, and salt in a large basin.
2. In a separate bowl, whisk together milk, vegetable oil, and eggs.

3. The wet ingredients are poured into the dry ingredients and stirred until just combined.
4. Preheat the waffle iron and pour the batter onto it, spreading it evenly.
5. Cook until golden brown and crisp.

Nutritional Values (per serving):
Calories: 320 | Fat: 15g | Protein: 8g |
Carbs: 40g | Fiber: 2g | Sugar: 5g |
Sodium: 450mg

Breakfast Burrito

Ingredients:
- 4 large eggs
- 1/2 cup washed and drained black beans
- 1/4 cup diced tomatoes
- 1/4 cup shredded cheese
- 2 large tortillas

Directions:
1. Crack 4 eggs into a bowl, whisk, and scramble in a heated skillet until fully cooked.
2. Mix in black beans, diced tomatoes, and shredded cheese.
3. Warm tortillas in the skillet or microwave.
4. Spoon the egg mixture onto each tortilla, roll into burritos, and serve.

Nutritional Values (per serving):
Calories: 380 | Fat: 20g | Protein: 18g |
Carbs: 30g | Fiber: 5g | Sugar: 2g |
Sodium: 550mg

Crispy Baked Tofu

Prep Time: 10 minutes | Baking Time: 25 minutes | Servings: 4

Ingredients:
- 1 block diced, pressed, extra-firm tofu
- 2 tbsp soy sauce
- 1 tbsp olive oil
- 1 tsp garlic powder
- 1 tsp smoked paprika

Directions:
1. Before beginning, preheat the oven to 400°F (200°C) and prepare a baking sheet with parchment paper.
2. In a bowl, toss tofu cubes with soy sauce, olive oil, garlic powder, and smoked paprika.
3. Spread the tofu on the prepared baking sheet in a single layer.
4. Bake for 25 minutes, flipping the tofu halfway through until it becomes crispy and golden.

Nutritional Values (per serving):
Calories: 150 | Fat: 8g | Protein: 12g |
Carbs: 10g | Fiber: 2g | Sugar: 1g |
Sodium: 300mg

Chickpea Scramble Bowl

Prep Time: 15 minutes | Cooking Time: 10 minutes | Servings: 3

Ingredients:
- 1 can chickpeas, drained and rinsed
- 1 tsp olive oil
- 1/2 onion, diced
- 1 bell pepper, diced
- 1 tsp cumin
- Salt and pepper to taste

Directions:
1. Heat the olive oil in a pan over medium heat.
2. Add diced onion and bell pepper, sauté until softened.
3. Add chickpeas, cumin, salt, and pepper. Cook until chickpeas are heated through.
4. Serve in bowls and enjoy.

Nutritional Values (per serving):
Calories: 220 | Fat: 5g | Protein: 8g |
Carbs: 35g | Fiber: 8g | Sugar: 6g |
Sodium: 400mg

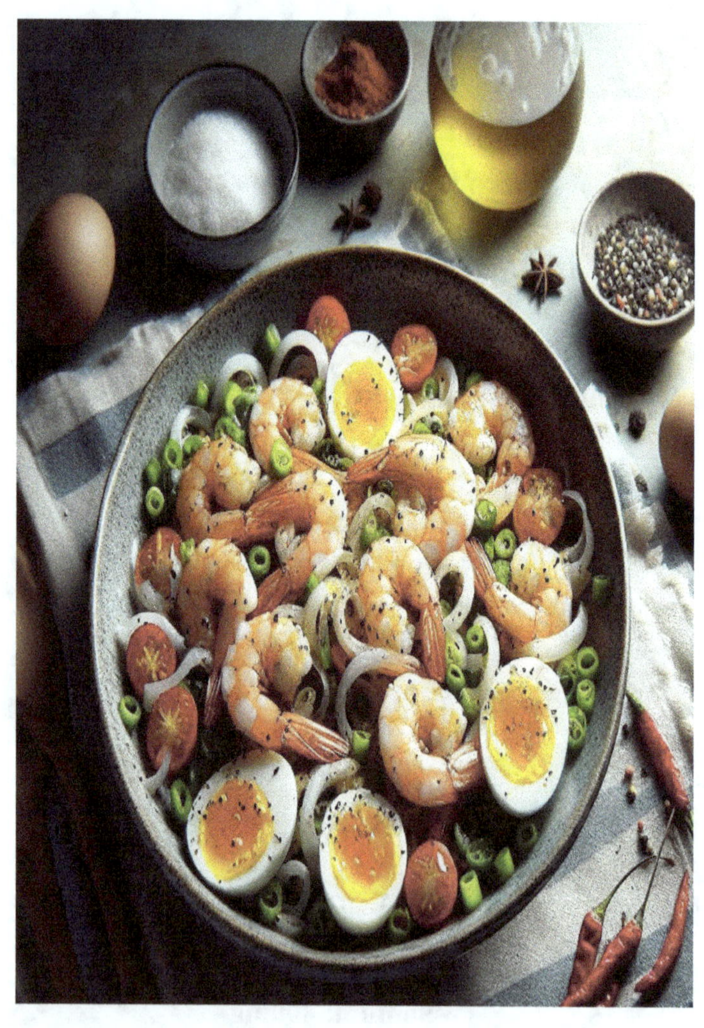

Chapter 4: Lunch Recipes

Coconut Veggie Wraps

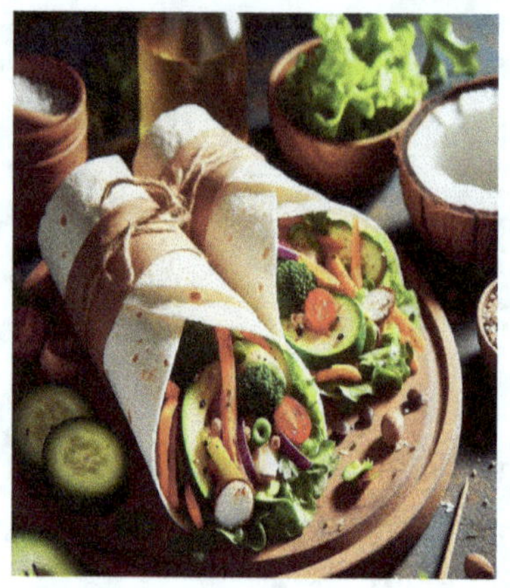

Preparation Time: 20 minutes
Cooking Time: 10 minutes
Servings: 2

Ingredients:
- 4 large whole-grain tortillas
- 1 cup coconut rice, cooked
- 1 cup mixed veggies (bell peppers, carrots, zucchini), sliced
- 1/2 cup shredded coconut, toasted
- 1/4 cup fresh cilantro, chopped

Directions:
1. Cook 1 cup of whole-grain rice with coconut milk according to package instructions.
2. Toast shredded coconut in a dry pan until golden brown.

3. Warm tortillas and assemble with cooked coconut rice, mixed veggies, toasted shredded coconut, and chopped cilantro.
4. Roll tightly and slice in half before serving.

Nutritional Values (per serving):
Calories: 400 | Fat: 15g | Protein: 8g |
Carbs: 60g | Fiber: 8g | Sugar: 3g |
Sodium: 350mg

One-Pan Halibut

Prep Time: 15 minutes | Baking Time: 20 minutes | Servings: 2

Ingredients:
- 2 halibut fillets
- 1 lemon, sliced
- 2 tbsp olive oil
- 1 tsp garlic powder
- Salt and pepper to taste

Directions:
1. Preheat the oven to 375°F (190°C).
2. Place halibut fillets on a baking sheet.
3. Drizzle olive oil over the fillets, then season with garlic powder, salt, and pepper.
4. Top each fillet with lemon slices.
5. Bake in the preheated oven for about 20 minutes or until the fish flakes easily with a fork.

Nutritional Values (per serving):
Calories: 250 | Fat: 12g | Protein: 30g |
Carbs: 2g | Fiber: 1g | Sugar: 0g |
Sodium: 400mg

Balsamic-Glazed Roasted Cauliflower

Prep Time: 10 minutes | Roasting Time: 25 minutes | Servings: 4

Ingredients:
- 1 head cauliflower, cut into florets
- 2 tbsp olive oil
- 3 tbsp balsamic vinegar
- 1 tsp honey
- Salt and pepper to taste

Directions:
1. Preheat the oven to 400°F (200°C).
2. Toss cauliflower florets in olive oil, balsamic vinegar, honey, salt, and pepper.
3. Spread cauliflower on a baking sheet in a single layer.
4. Roast for 25 minutes or until golden brown and tender, stirring halfway through.

Nutritional Values (per serving):
Calories: 120 | Fat: 7g | Protein: 3g |
Carbs: 14g | Fiber: 5g | Sugar: 7g |
Sodium: 100mg

Lentil Rice Soup

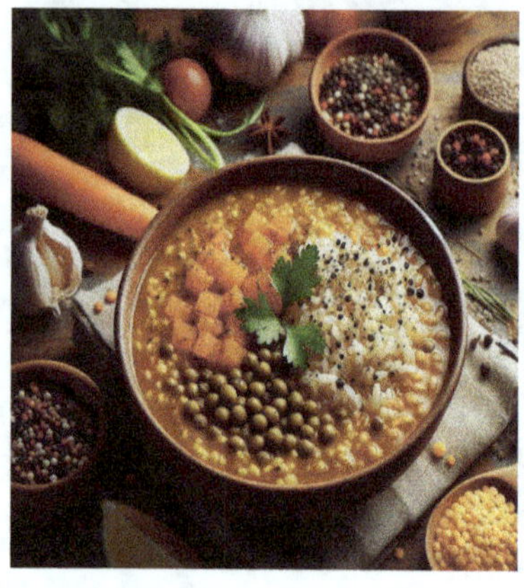

Preparation Time: 15 minutes
Cooking Time: 30 minutes
Servings: 6

Ingredients:
- 1 cup lentils, rinsed
- 1 cup brown rice, cooked
- 1 onion, chopped
- 2 carrots, diced
- 2 celery stalks, sliced
- 4 cups vegetable broth
- 1 can diced tomatoes
- 1 tsp cumin
- Salt and pepper to taste

Directions:
1. Rinse 1 cup of lentils under cold water.

2. In a large pot, sauté chopped onion, diced carrots, and sliced celery until softened.

3. Add lentils, cooked brown rice, vegetable broth, diced tomatoes, cumin, salt, and pepper. Simmer until lentils are tender.

4. Adjust seasoning as needed and serve hot.

Nutritional Values (per serving):
Calories: 280 | Fat: 1g | Protein: 15g |
Carbs: 55g | Fiber: 12g | Sugar: 5g |
Sodium: 700mg

Turkey with Barley and Squash

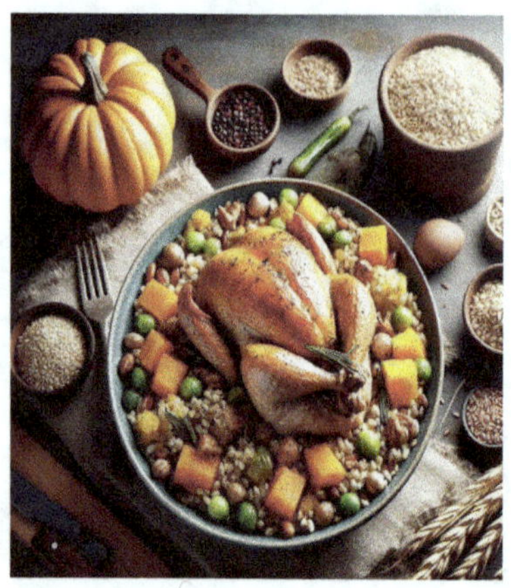

Preparation Time: 20 minutes
Cooking Time: 30 minutes
Servings: 4

Ingredients:
- 1 lb turkey breast, diced
- 1 cup barley, cooked
- 2 cups butternut squash, diced
- 1 onion, chopped
- 2 cloves garlic, minced
- 2 tbsp olive oil
- 1 tsp thyme
- Salt and pepper to taste

Directions:
1. Heat the olive oil in a big skillet over medium heat.
2. Add diced turkey and cook until browned.

3. Add chopped onion and minced garlic, sauté until softened.

4. Stir in diced butternut squash, cooked barley, thyme, salt, and pepper.

5. Cook until the squash is tender. Serve hot.

Nutritional Values (per serving):
Calories: 350 | Fat: 8g | Protein: 30g |
Carbs: 40g | Fiber: 8g | Sugar: 3g |
Sodium: 400mg

Salmon Salad Niçoise

Prep Time: 15 minutes | Cooking Time: 10 minutes | Servings: 2

Ingredients:
- 2 salmon fillets
- 4 cups mixed greens
- 1 cup cherry tomatoes, halved
- 1/2 cup olives, sliced
- 2 hard-boiled eggs, sliced
- 1/4 cup green beans, blanched

Directions:

1. Season salmon fillets with salt and pepper and cook until flaky.

2. In a large bowl, arrange mixed greens and top with cherry tomatoes, sliced olives, hard-boiled egg slices, and blanched green beans.

3. Place cooked salmon on top. After adding a drizzle of your preferred dressing, serve.

Nutritional Values (per serving):
Calories: 400 | Fat: 20g | Protein: 35g |
Carbs: 20g | Fiber: 6g | Sugar: 4g |
Sodium: 500mg

Egg Fried Rice

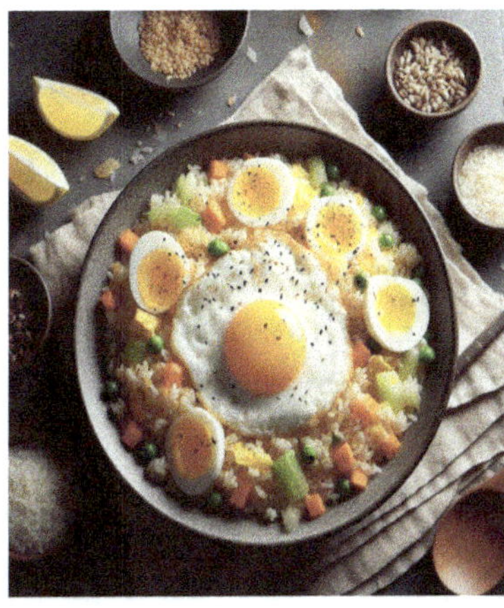

Preparation Time: 15 minutes
Cooking Time: 10 minutes
Servings: 3

Ingredients:
- 3 cups cooked jasmine rice, cooled
- 3 eggs, beaten
- 1 cup mixed vegetables (peas, carrots, corn)
- 2 green onions, sliced
- 2 tbsp soy sauce
- 1 tbsp sesame oil
- 1 tbsp vegetable oil

Directions:
1. Heat vegetable oil in a wok or large skillet over medium heat.
2. Add beaten eggs and scramble until just cooked. Remove from the wok.

3. Stir-fry mixed vegetables until tender.

4. Add cooked rice and scrambled eggs back to the wok. Add sesame oil and soy sauce and stir.

5. Garnish with sliced green onions and serve hot.

Nutritional Values (per serving):
Calories: 300 | Fat: 10g | Protein: 10g |
Carbs: 40g | Fiber: 3g | Sugar: 2g |
Sodium: 800mg

Spinach And Eggs Salad

Prep Time: 15 minutes | Cooking Time: 5 minutes | Servings: 2

Ingredients:
- 4 cups fresh spinach
- 4 eggs, poached
- 1/2 cup cherry tomatoes, halved
- 1/4 cup feta cheese, crumbled
- 1/4 cup balsamic vinaigrette dressing

Directions:
1. Divide fresh spinach between two plates.
2. Top with poached eggs, halved cherry tomatoes, and crumbled feta cheese.
3. Drizzle with balsamic vinaigrette dressing before serving.

Nutritional Values (per serving):
Calories: 250 | Fat: 15g | Protein: 15g | Carbs: 15g | Fiber: 4g | Sugar: 6g | Sodium: 500mg

Sardines with Artichokes and Greens

Prep Time: 15 minutes | Cooking Time: 10 minutes | Servings: 2

Ingredients:
- 1 can sardines in olive oil
- 1 cup washed and quartered artichoke hearts
- 4 cups mixed greens
- 1 lemon, juiced
- Salt and pepper to taste

Directions:
1. In a large bowl, combine mixed greens, quartered artichoke hearts, and sardines.
2. Drizzle with lemon juice and season with salt and pepper.
3. Toss gently and serve immediately.

Nutritional Values (per serving):
Calories: 300 | Fat: 20g | Protein: 20g | Carbs: 10g | Fiber: 5g | Sugar: 3g | Sodium: 600mg

---

Asian-Inspired Peanut Noodles

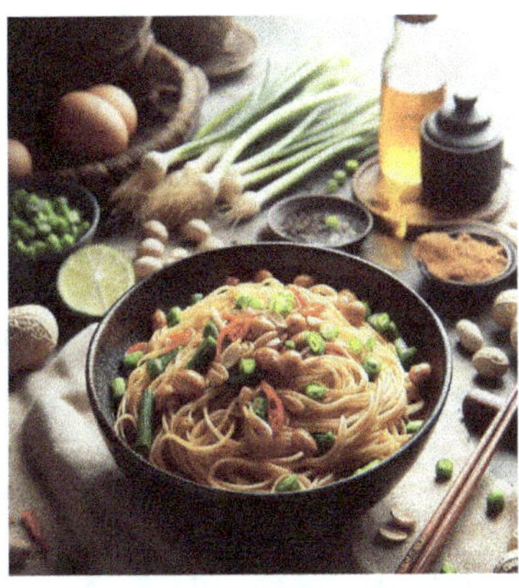

Preparation Time: 15 minutes
Cooking Time: 10 minutes
Servings: 4

Ingredients:
- 8 oz rice noodles, cooked
- 1/2 cup peanut butter
- 1/4 cup soy sauce
- 2 tbsp sesame oil
- 1 tbsp rice vinegar
- 1 tbsp honey
- 1 tsp ginger, grated
- 2 cloves garlic, minced
- 1 cup shredded carrots
- 1/4 cup chopped green onions
- Sesame seeds for garnish

Directions:

1. In a bowl, whisk together peanut butter, soy sauce, sesame oil, rice vinegar, honey, grated ginger, and minced garlic.

2. Toss cooked rice noodles in the sauce until well coated.

3. Add shredded carrots and chopped green onions. Mix gently.

4. Garnish with sesame seeds before serving.

Nutritional Values (per serving):
Calories: 400 | Fat: 20g | Protein: 10g |
Carbs: 45g | Fiber: 5g | Sugar: 8g |
Sodium: 600mg

Chapter 5: Dinner Recipes

Bok Choy and Chicken Stir-Fry

Preparation Time: 15 minutes
Cooking Time: 15 minutes
Servings: 4

Ingredients:
- 1 lb chicken breast, thinly sliced
- 4 baby bok choy, chopped
- 1 bell pepper, sliced
- 1 cup snow peas
- 3 tbsp soy sauce
- 1 tbsp oyster sauce
- 1 tbsp sesame oil
- 2 cloves garlic, minced
- 1 tsp ginger, grated
- Cooked rice for serving

Directions:
1. Heat the sesame oil in a wok or big pan over medium-high heat.
2. Add sliced chicken and stir-fry until browned and cooked through.
3. Add minced garlic and grated ginger, stir for 1 minute.

4. Add chopped bok choy, bell pepper, and snow peas. Stir-fry until vegetables are tender-crisp.

5. Mix in soy sauce and oyster sauce. Stir to combine.

6. Serve the stir-fry over cooked rice.

Nutritional Values (per serving):
Calories: 350 | Fat: 12g | Protein: 30g |
Carbs: 25g | Fiber: 6g | Sugar: 4g |
Sodium: 800mg

Red Beans and Rice

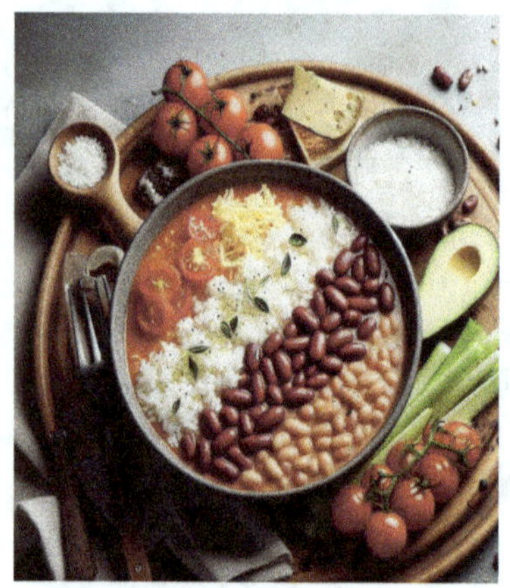

Preparation Time: 15 minutes
Cooking Time: 30 minutes
Servings: 6

Ingredients:
- 2 cups cooked red beans
- 2 cups cooked rice
- 1 onion, chopped
- 1 bell pepper, chopped
- 2 celery stalks, diced
- 3 cloves garlic, minced
- 1 tsp thyme
- 1 tsp smoked paprika
- Salt and pepper to taste

Directions:

1. In a large pot, sauté chopped onion, bell pepper, celery, and minced garlic until softened.

2. Add cooked red beans, thyme, smoked paprika, salt, and pepper. Stir to combine.

3. Let the mixture simmer for at least 20-25 minutes, allowing flavors to meld.

4. Serve over cooked rice.

Nutritional Values (per serving):
Calories: 300 | Fat: 1g | Protein: 10g |
Carbs: 60g | Fiber: 10g | Sugar: 3g |
Sodium: 500mg

Black Bean Stuffed Sweet Potatoes

Preparation Time: 10 minutes
Baking Time: 45 minutes
Servings: 4

Ingredients:
- 4 medium sweet potatoes
- 1 can black beans, drained and rinsed
- 1 cup fresh or frozen corn kernels
- 1 cup cherry tomatoes, halved
- 1/2 cup red onion, finely chopped
- 1/4 cup cilantro, chopped
- 1 avocado, sliced
- Lime wedges for serving

Directions:
1. Preheat the oven to 400°F (200°C).
2. Prick sweet potatoes with a fork and bake for 45 minutes or until tender.
3. In a bowl, combine black beans, corn, cherry tomatoes, red onion, and cilantro.
4. Cut a slit in each sweet potato and fluff the insides with a fork.

5. Stuff each sweet potato with the black bean mixture.

6. Top with sliced avocado and serve with lime wedges.

Mushroom and Spinach Lasagna

Preparation Time: 30 minutes
Baking Time: 40 minutes
Servings: 8

Ingredients:
- 9 lasagna noodles, cooked
- 1 lb mushrooms, sliced
- 4 cups fresh spinach
- 2 cups ricotta cheese
- 2 cups mozzarella cheese, shredded
- 1 cup Parmesan cheese, grated
- 2 cups marinara sauce
- 2 cloves garlic, minced
- 1 tsp dried oregano
- Salt and pepper to taste

Directions:
1. Preheat the oven to 375°F (190°C).
2. In a pan, sauté sliced mushrooms and minced garlic until mushrooms release their moisture.
3. Add fresh spinach and cook until wilted. Season with oregano, salt, and pepper.
4. In a bowl, mix ricotta cheese with half of the mozzarella and Parmesan cheeses.

5. In a baking dish, layer marinara sauce, lasagna noodles, ricotta mixture, and mushroom-spinach mixture.

6. Repeat layers, finishing with a layer of marinara sauce on top. Sprinkle remaining cheese on the top layer.

7. Bake for 40 minutes or until bubbly and golden.

Nutritional Values (per serving):
Calories: 450 | Fat: 20g | Protein: 25g |
Carbs: 40g | Fiber: 5g | Sugar: 7g |
Sodium: 700mg

Tuna Vegetable Wrap

Preparation Time: 10 minutes | Servings: 2

Ingredients:
- 1 can tuna, drained
- 1/2 cup Greek yogurt
- 1/4 cup red onion, finely chopped
- 1/4 cup celery, finely chopped
- 1/4 cup cucumber, diced
- 2 tbsp mayonnaise
- 2 whole-grain wraps

Directions:
1. In a bowl, mix drained tuna, Greek yogurt, red onion, celery, cucumber, and mayonnaise.
2. Lay out the whole-grain wraps and evenly distribute the tuna mixture on each.
3. Roll the wraps tightly, cut in half, and serve.

Nutritional Values (per serving):
Calories: 350 | Fat: 15g | Protein: 25g |
Carbs: 30g | Fiber: 5g | Sugar: 5g |
Sodium: 600mg

Spaghetti With Chickpeas Meatballs

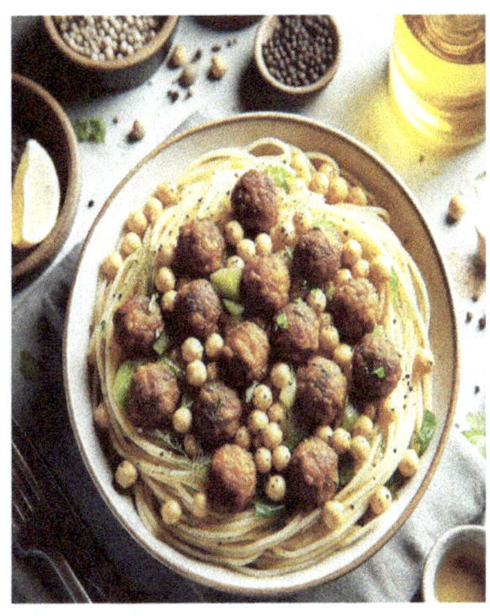

Preparation Time: 20 minutes
Cooking Time: 25 minutes
Servings: 4

Ingredients:
- 8 oz spaghetti, cooked
- 1 can chickpeas, drained and mashed
- 1/2 cup breadcrumbs
- 1/4 cup grated Parmesan cheese
- 1/4 cup fresh parsley, chopped
- 2 cloves garlic, minced
- 1 egg
- Salt and pepper to taste
- Marinara sauce for serving

Directions:

1. In a bowl, combine mashed chickpeas, breadcrumbs, Parmesan cheese, chopped parsley, minced garlic, egg, salt, and pepper.

2. Form the mixture into meatballs and bake in the oven at 375°F (190°C) for 20 minutes.

3. Cook spaghetti according to package instructions.

4. Serve chickpea meatballs over cooked spaghetti with marinara sauce.

Nutritional Values (per serving):
Calories: 400 | Fat: 10g | Protein: 15g |
Carbs: 60g | Fiber: 8g | Sugar: 4g |
Sodium: 700mg

Lentil Bolognese

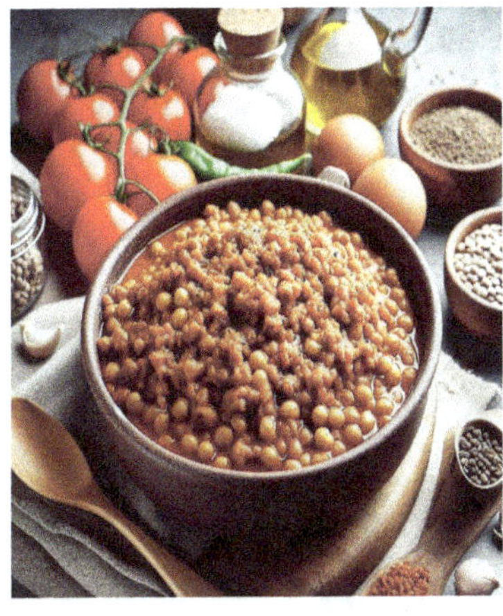

Preparation Time: 15 minutes
Cooking Time: 30 minutes
Servings: 6

Ingredients:
- 2 cups cooked lentils
- 1 onion, chopped
- 2 carrots, diced
- 2 celery stalks, sliced
- 3 cloves garlic, minced
- 1 can crushed tomatoes
- 1/4 cup tomato paste
- 1 tsp dried oregano
- 1 tsp dried basil
- Salt and pepper to taste
- 8 oz whole-grain spaghetti, cooked

Directions:

1. In a large pot, sauté chopped onion, diced carrots, sliced celery, and minced garlic until softened.

2. Add cooked lentils, crushed tomatoes, tomato paste, oregano, basil, salt, and pepper. Simmer for 20-25 minutes.

3. Serve over cooked whole-grain spaghetti.

Nutritional Values (per serving):
Calories: 350 | Fat: 5g | Protein: 15g |
Carbs: 65g | Fiber: 12g | Sugar: 8g |
Sodium: 500mg

Shrimp And Asparagus Salad

Prep Time: 15 minutes | Cooking Time: 5 minutes | Servings: 2

Ingredients:
- 8 oz shrimp, peeled and deveined
- 1 bunch asparagus, trimmed and blanched
- 4 cups mixed salad greens
- 1/4 cup cherry tomatoes, halved
- 1/4 cup feta cheese, crumbled
- 1/4 cup balsamic vinaigrette dressing

Directions:
1. In a pan, cook shrimp until pink and opaque.
2. In a large bowl, combine blanched asparagus, mixed salad greens, cherry tomatoes, and cooked shrimp.
3. Top with crumbled feta cheese and drizzle with balsamic vinaigrette dressing.
4. Toss gently and serve.

Nutritional Values (per serving):
Calories: 300 | Fat: 15g | Protein: 25g | Carbs: 15g | Fiber: 5g | Sugar: 8g | Sodium: 600mg

Veggie Burger with Avocado

Prep Time: 20 minutes | Cooking Time: 10 minutes | Servings: 4

Ingredients:
- 4 veggie burger patties
- 4 whole-grain burger buns
- 1 avocado, sliced
- 1 cup mixed greens
- 1/4 cup red onion, thinly sliced
- 1/4 cup hummus

Directions:
1. Cook veggie burger patties according to package instructions.
2. Toast whole-grain burger buns.
3. Assemble burgers with veggie patties, sliced avocado, mixed greens, thinly sliced red onion, and a dollop of hummus.
4. Serve immediately.

Nutritional Values (per serving):
Calories: 400 | Fat: 15g | Protein: 20g |
Carbs: 50g | Fiber: 10g | Sugar: 5g |
Sodium: 600mg

Broccoli and Cheddar Soup

Preparation Time: 15 minutes
Cooking Time: 25 minutes
Servings: 6

Ingredients:
- 1 lb broccoli, chopped
- 1 onion, chopped
- 2 carrots, diced
- 2 cloves garlic, minced
- 4 cups vegetable broth
- 2 cups shredded cheddar cheese
- 1 cup milk
- 2 tbsp butter
- 3 tbsp all-purpose flour
- Salt and pepper to taste

Directions:
1. In a pot, sauté chopped onion, diced carrots, and minced garlic in butter until softened.
2. Add chopped broccoli and vegetable broth. Simmer until vegetables are tender.
3. In a separate saucepan, whisk flour into milk over medium heat until thickened.

4. Add the milk mixture to the soup, stirring well.
Bring to a gentle boil.
5. Reduce heat, stir in shredded cheddar cheese until
melted. Season with salt and pepper.
6. Serve hot.

Nutritional Values (per serving):
Calories: 350 | Fat: 20g | Protein: 15g |
Carbs: 30g | Fiber: 6g | Sugar: 8g |
Sodium: 800mg

Chapter 6: Snacks/Desserts

Simple Banana Cookies

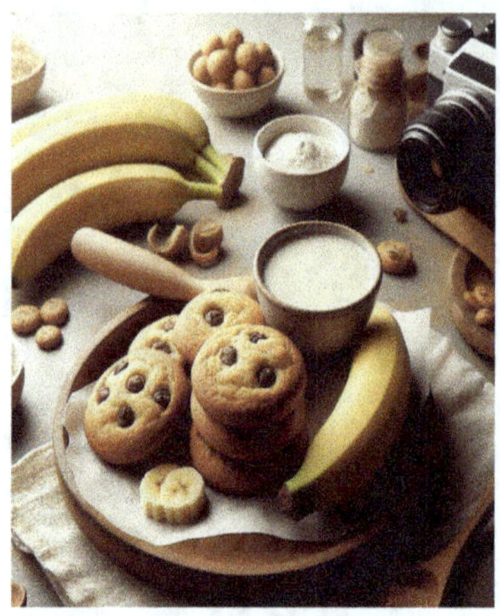

Preparation Time: 10 minutes

Baking Time: 12 minutes

Servings: 12 cookies

Ingredients:
- 3 ripe bananas, mashed
- 2 cups rolled oats
- 1/4 cup almond butter
- 1/4 cup honey
- 1 tsp vanilla extract
- 1/2 tsp cinnamon
- Pinch of salt

Directions:

1. Before beginning, preheat the oven to 350°F (180°C) and prepare a baking sheet with parchment paper.

2. In a bowl, combine mashed bananas, rolled oats, almond butter, honey, vanilla extract, cinnamon, and a pinch of salt.

3. Drop spoonfuls of the mixture onto the prepared baking sheet.

4. Bake for 12 minutes, or until well-browned.

5. Allow to cool before serving.

Nutritional Values (per serving - 1 cookie):
Calories: 120 | Fat: 4g | Protein: 3g |
Carbs: 20g | Fiber: 3g | Sugar: 8g |
Sodium: 10mg

Roasted Walnuts

Prep Time: 5 minutes | Roasting Time: 10 minutes | Servings: 1 cup

Ingredients:
- 1 cup walnuts
- 1 tbsp olive oil
- 1/2 tsp salt
- 1/2 tsp paprika

Directions:
1. Preheat the oven to 350°F (180°C).
2. In a bowl, toss walnuts with olive oil, salt, and paprika.
3. Spread the walnuts in a single layer on a baking sheet.
4. Roast for 10 minutes, stirring halfway through.
5. Allow to cool before serving.

Nutritional Values (per serving - 1/4 cup):
Calories: 200 | Fat: 20g | Protein: 5g |
Carbs: 4g | Fiber: 2g | Sugar: 1g |
Sodium: 290mg

Dark Chocolate Bites

Prep Time: 15 minutes | Chilling Time: 1 hour |
Servings: 12 bites

Ingredients:
- 1 cup dark chocolate chips
- 1/4 cup almonds, chopped
- 1/4 cup dried cranberries
- Sea salt for sprinkling

Directions:
1. Melt dark chocolate chips in a heatproof bowl over a pot of simmering water or in the microwave.
2. Mix in chopped almonds and dried cranberries.
3. Spoon small portions onto a parchment-lined tray.
4. Sprinkle with sea salt and refrigerate for at least 1 hour.
5. Once set, break into bite-sized pieces.

Nutritional Values (per serving - 1 bite):
Calories: 80 | Fat: 5g | Protein: 1g |
Carbs: 10g | Fiber: 2g | Sugar: 6g |
Sodium: 5mg

Baked Carrot Chips

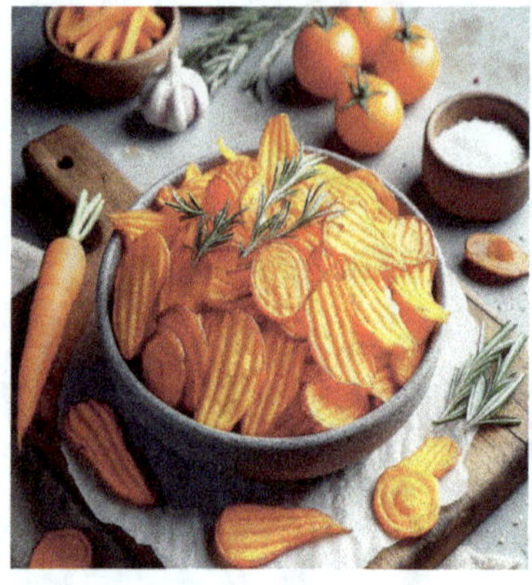

Preparation Time: 10 minutes
Baking Time: 20 minutes
Servings: 2 cups

Ingredients:
- 4 large carrots, peeled and thinly sliced
- 1 tbsp olive oil
- 1/2 tsp smoked paprika
- 1/2 tsp garlic powder
- Salt and pepper to taste

Directions:

1. Before beginning, preheat the oven to 400°F (200°C) and prepare a baking sheet with parchment paper.

2. Toss thinly sliced carrots with olive oil, smoked paprika, garlic powder, salt, and pepper.

3. Arrange in a single layer on the prepared baking sheet.

4. Bake for 20 minutes or until crisp, flipping halfway through.

5. Allow to cool before serving.

Nutritional Values (per serving - 1/2 cup):
Calories: 60 | Fat: 3g | Protein: 1g |
Carbs: 8g | Fiber: 2g | Sugar: 4g |
Sodium: 30mg

Spicy Nut Mix

Prep Time: 5 minutes | Roasting Time: 10 minutes | Servings: 2 cups

Ingredients:
- 1 cup mixed nuts (walnuts, cashews, and almonds)
- 1 tbsp olive oil
- 1 tsp chili powder
- 1/2 tsp cayenne pepper
- 1/2 tsp cumin
- Salt to taste

Directions:
1. Before beginning, preheat the oven to 350°F (180°C) and prepare a baking sheet with parchment paper.
2. In a bowl, toss mixed nuts with olive oil, chili powder, cayenne pepper, cumin, and salt.
3. Spread the nut mixture in a single layer on the prepared baking sheet.
4. Roast for 10 minutes, stirring halfway through.
5. Allow to cool before serving.

Nutritional Values (per serving - 1/4 cup):
Calories: 150 | Fat: 13g | Protein: 4g |
Carbs: 6g | Fiber: 2g | Sugar: 1g |
Sodium: 50mg

Yogurt Parfait

Preparation Time: 10 minutes | Servings: 2

Ingredients:
- 2 cups Greek yogurt
- 1 cup granola
- 1 cup mixed berries (raspberries, strawberries, blueberries, etc)
- 2 tbsp honey

Directions:
1. In serving glasses or bowls, layer Greek yogurt, granola, and mixed berries.
2. Repeat the layers until the glass is filled.
3. Drizzle honey on top.
4. Serve immediately and enjoy!

Nutritional Values (per serving):
Calories: 350 | Fat: 10g | Protein: 20g |
Carbs: 45g | Fiber: 6g | Sugar: 20g |
Sodium: 100mg

Hummus

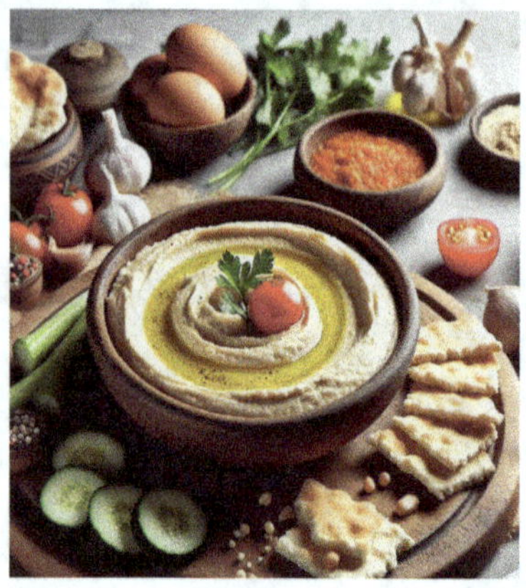

**Preparation Time:
10 minutes
Servings: 2 cups**

Ingredients:
- 1 can chickpeas, drained and rinsed
- 1/4 cup tahini
- 2 cloves garlic, minced
- 2 tbsp lemon juice
- 2 tbsp olive oil
- 1/2 tsp cumin
- Salt and pepper to taste
- Water (as needed for consistency)

Directions:

1. In a food processor, combine chickpeas, tahini, minced garlic, lemon juice, olive oil, cumin, salt, and pepper.

2. Blend until smooth, adding water as needed for desired consistency.

3. Transfer to a bowl and serve with pita bread or vegetable sticks.

Nutritional Values (per serving - 2 tbsp):
Calories: 50 | Fat: 4g | Protein: 2g |
Carbs: 3g | Fiber: 1g | Sugar: 0g |
Sodium: 50mg

Roasted Chickpeas

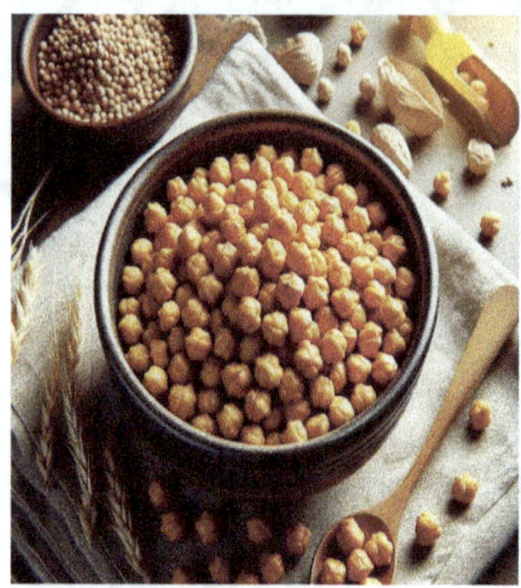

Preparation Time: 5 minutes
Roasting Time: 25 minutes
Servings: 2 cups

Ingredients:
- 2 cans chickpeas, drained and dried
- 2 tbsp olive oil
- 1 tsp smoked paprika
- 1/2 tsp cumin
- 1/2 tsp garlic powder
- Salt to taste

Directions:

1. Before beginning, preheat the oven to 400°F (200°C) and prepare a baking sheet with parchment paper.

2. In a bowl, toss chickpeas with olive oil, smoked paprika, cumin, garlic powder, and salt.

3. Arrange the chickpeas on the baking sheet that has been preheated in a single layer.

4. Roast for 25 minutes or until crispy, stirring halfway through.

5. Allow to cool before serving.

Nutritional Values (per serving - 1/4 cup):
Calories: 50 | Fat: 2g | Protein: 2g |
Carbs: 6g | Fiber: 2g | Sugar: 0g |
Sodium: 100mg

Potato Chips

Prep Time: 15 minutes | Baking Time: 20 minutes | Servings: 2 cups

Ingredients:
- 2 large potatoes, thinly sliced
- 2 tbsp olive oil
- 1 tsp paprika
- 1/2 tsp garlic powder
- Salt to taste

Directions:
1. Before beginning, preheat the oven to 400°F (200°C) and prepare a baking sheet with parchment paper.
2. In a bowl, toss thinly sliced potatoes with olive oil, paprika, garlic powder, and salt.
3. Arrange the potato slices in a single layer on the prepared baking sheet.
4. Bake for 20 minutes or until golden and crispy, flipping halfway through.
5. Allow to cool before serving.

Nutritional Values (per serving - 1/2 cup):
Calories: 120 | Fat: 5g | Protein: 2g |
Carbs: 18g | Fiber: 2g | Sugar: 1g |
Sodium: 100mg

Carrot Cupcakes

Preparation Time: 20 minutes
Baking Time: 18 minutes
Servings: 12 cupcakes

Ingredients:
- 1½ cups grated carrots
- 1 cup all-purpose flour
- 1/2 cup whole wheat flour
- 1/2 cup brown sugar
- 1/4 cup coconut oil, melted
- 2 eggs
- 1/2 cup unsweetened applesauce
- 1 tsp baking powder
- 1/2 tsp baking soda
- 1/2 tsp cinnamon
- 1/4 tsp salt
- 1/2 cup chopped walnuts (optional)
- Cream cheese frosting (optional)

Directions:

1. Preheat the oven to 350°F (180°C) and line a muffin tin with cupcake liners.

2. In a bowl, whisk together grated carrots, all-purpose flour, whole wheat flour, brown sugar,

melted coconut oil, eggs, applesauce, baking powder, baking soda, cinnamon, and salt.

3. Fold in chopped walnuts if desired.

4. Spoon the batter into cupcake liners, filling each about 2/3 full.

5. Bake for 18 minutes, or until a toothpick inserted into the centre comes out clean.

6. Allow to cool before frosting, if desired.

Nutritional Values (per serving - 1 cupcake without frosting):
Calories: 150 | Fat: 7g | Protein: 3g |
Carbs: 20g | Fiber: 2g | Sugar: 8g |
Sodium: 120mg

Chapter 7: Smoothie Recipes

Peanut Butter and Chocolate Smoothie

Preparation Time: 5 minutes | Servings: 2

Ingredients:
- 2 ripe bananas
- 2 tbsp peanut butter
- 2 tbsp cocoa powder
- 1 cup Greek yogurt
- 1 cup almond milk
- 1 tbsp honey (optional)

Directions:
1. In a blender, combine ripe bananas, peanut butter, cocoa powder, Greek yogurt, almond milk, and honey.
2. Blend until smooth and creamy.
3. Pour into glasses and enjoy!

Nutritional Values (per serving):
Calories: 300 | Fat: 12g | Protein: 15g |
Carbs: 40g | Fiber: 6g | Sugar: 20g |
Sodium: 150mg

Tropical Flaxseed Smoothie

Preparation Time: 5 minutes | Servings: 2

Ingredients:
- 1 cup mango chunks (fresh or frozen)
- 1 cup (fresh or frozen) pineapple chunks
- 1 banana
- 1 tbsp flaxseeds
- 1 cup coconut water
- Ice cubes (optional)

Directions:
1. In a blender, combine mango chunks, pineapple chunks, banana, flaxseeds, coconut water, and ice cubes if desired.
2. Blend until smooth.
3. Pour into glasses and enjoy the tropical goodness!

Nutritional Values (per serving):
Calories: 200 | Fat: 3g | Protein: 3g |
Carbs: 45g | Fiber: 8g | Sugar: 30g |
Sodium: 50mg

Mixed Berry Smoothie

Preparation Time: 5 minutes | Servings: 2

Ingredients:
- 1 cup mixed berries (blueberries, strawberries, and raspberries)
- 1 banana
- 1/2 cup Greek yogurt
- 1 cup almond milk
- 1 tbsp chia seeds
- 1 tsp honey (optional)

Directions:

1. In a blender, combine mixed berries, banana, Greek yogurt, almond milk, chia seeds, and honey if desired.
2. Blend until smooth and creamy.
3. Pour into glasses and savor the berry goodness!

Nutritional Values (per serving):
Calories: 250 | Fat: 8g | Protein: 10g |
Carbs: 40g | Fiber: 8g | Sugar: 20g |
Sodium: 120mg

Berry Avocado Smoothie

Ingredients:
- 1 cup mixed berries (blueberries, strawberries, and raspberries)
- 1/2 avocado, peeled and pitted
- 1 banana
- 1 cup spinach leaves
- 1 cup coconut water
- Ice cubes (optional)

Directions:
1. In a blender, combine mixed berries, avocado, banana, spinach leaves, coconut water, and ice cubes if desired.
2. Blend until smooth and green.
3. Pour into glasses and enjoy the nutritious blend!

Nutritional Values (per serving):
Calories: 200 | Fat: 9g | Protein: 4g |
Carbs: 30g | Fiber: 10g | Sugar: 15g |
Sodium: 50mg

Citrus Smoothie

Ingredients:
- 1 orange, peeled and segmented
- 1 grapefruit, peeled and segmented
- 1 banana
- 1/2 cup Greek yogurt
- 1 cup water
- Ice cubes (optional)

Directions:
1. In a blender, combine orange segments, grapefruit segments, banana, Greek yogurt, water, and ice cubes if desired.
2. Blend until citrusy and refreshing.
3. Pour into glasses and relish the zesty goodness!

Nutritional Values (per serving):
Calories: 180 | Fat: 1g | Protein: 6g |
Carbs: 40g | Fiber: 6g | Sugar: 25g |
Sodium: 30mg

Banana-Coconut Smoothie

Ingredients:
- 2 bananas
- 1/2 cup coconut milk
- 1/2 cup Greek yogurt
- 1/4 cup shredded coconut
- 1 tbsp chia seeds
- Ice cubes (optional)

Directions:

1. In a blender, combine bananas, coconut milk, Greek yogurt, shredded coconut, chia seeds, and ice cubes if desired.

2. Blend until smooth and creamy.

3. Pour into glasses and savor the tropical delight!

Nutritional Values (per serving):
Calories: 300 | Fat: 12g | Protein: 8g |
Carbs: 45g | Fiber: 7g | Sugar: 25g |
Sodium: 40mg

Cherry Berry Smoothie

Preparation Time: 5 minutes | Servings: 2

Ingredients:
- 1 cup mixed berries (cherries, blueberries, strawberries)
- 1/2 cup pomegranate juice
- 1/2 cup Greek yogurt
- 1 tbsp honey
- Ice cubes (optional)

Directions:
1. In a blender, combine mixed berries, pomegranate juice, Greek yogurt, honey, and ice cubes if desired.
2. Blend until smooth and vibrant.
3. Pour into glasses and enjoy the berry burst!

Nutritional Values (per serving):
Calories: 180 | Fat: 2g | Protein: 5g |
Carbs: 35g | Fiber: 5g | Sugar: 25g |
Sodium: 20mg

Mocha-Banana Smoothie

Preparation Time: 5 minutes | Servings: 2

Ingredients:
- 2 bananas
- 1 cup cold brew coffee
- 1/2 cup milk (dairy or plant-based)
- 2 tbsp cocoa powder
- 1 tbsp maple syrup
- Ice cubes (optional)

Directions:
1. In a blender, combine bananas, cold brew coffee, milk, cocoa powder, maple syrup, and ice cubes if desired.
2. Blend until smooth and caffeinated.
3. Pour into glasses and relish the mocha goodness!

Nutritional Values (per serving):
Calories: 150 | Fat: 2g | Protein: 3g |
Carbs: 30g | Fiber: 5g | Sugar: 15g |
Sodium: 20mg

Sweet Peach Smoothie

Preparation Time: 5 minutes | Servings: 2

Ingredients:
- 2 cups frozen peaches
- 1 banana
- 1/2 cup orange juice
- 1/2 cup Greek yogurt
- 1 tbsp honey
- Ice cubes (optional)

Directions:
1. In a blender, combine frozen peaches, banana, orange juice, Greek yogurt, honey, and ice cubes if desired.
2. Blend until smooth and peachy.
3. Pour into glasses and savor the sweet peach delight!

Nutritional Values (per serving):
Calories: 220 | Fat: 1g | Protein: 6g |
Carbs: 50g | Fiber: 6g | Sugar: 35g |
Sodium: 20mg

Spinach Kale Smoothie

Preparation Time: 5 minutes | Servings: 2

Ingredients:
- 1 cup spinach leaves
- 1 cup kale leaves, stems removed
- 1 banana
- 1/2 cup fresh or frozen pineapple chunks
- 1/2 cup orange juice
- 1/2 cup water
- 1 tbsp chia seeds
- Ice cubes (optional)

Directions:

1. In a blender, combine spinach leaves, kale leaves, banana, pineapple chunks, orange juice, water, chia seeds, and ice cubes if desired.

2. Blend until smooth and green.

3. Pour into glasses and enjoy the nutrient-packed goodness!

Nutritional Values (per serving):
Calories: 150 | Fat: 3g | Protein: 5g |
Carbs: 30g | Fiber: 8g | Sugar: 15g |
Sodium: 20mg

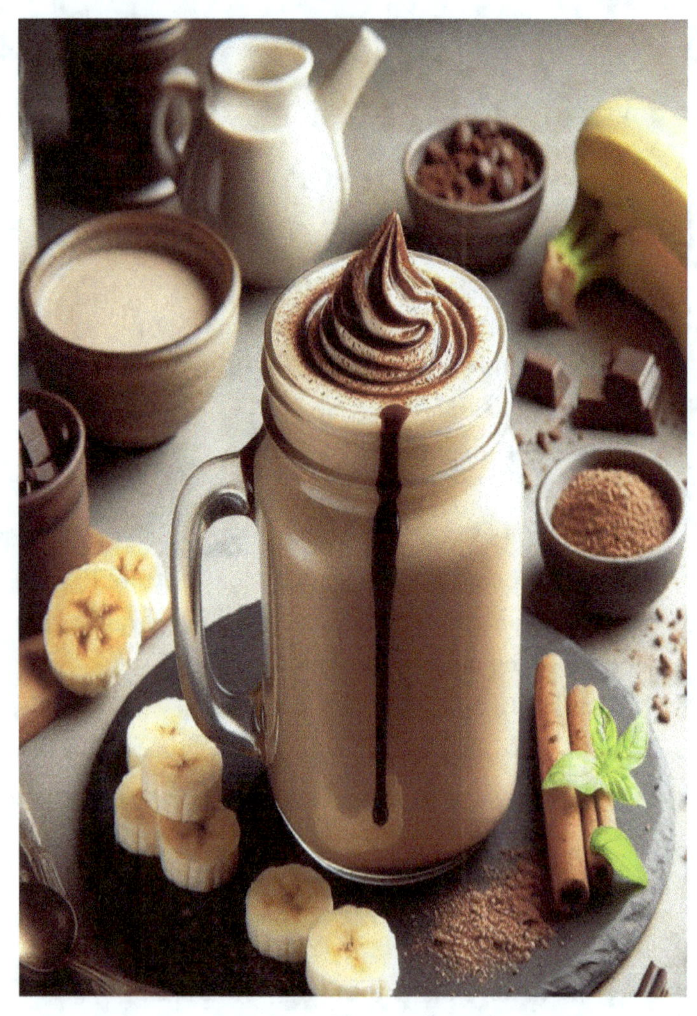

21-Day Meal Plan

Day 1:
Breakfast: Shrimp and Eggs Mix
Lunch: Coconut Veggie Wraps
Dinner: Bok Choy and Chicken Stir-Fry
Snacks/Desserts: Simple Banana Cookies

Day 2:
Breakfast: Savory Breakfast Sandwich
Lunch: One-Pan Halibut
Dinner: Red Beans and Rice
Snacks/Desserts: Roasted Walnuts

Day 3:
Breakfast: Almond Quinoa
Lunch: Balsamic-Glazed Roasted Cauliflower
Dinner: Black Bean Stuffed Sweet Potatoes
Snacks/Desserts: Dark Chocolate Bites

Day 4:
Breakfast: Coconut Buckwheat Porridge
Lunch: Lentil Rice Soup
Dinner: Mushroom and Spinach Lasagna
Snacks/Desserts: Baked Carrot Chips

Day 5:

Breakfast: Mixed Berry Smoothie
Lunch: Turkey with Barley and Squash
Dinner: Tuna Vegetable Wrap
Snacks/Desserts: Spicy Nut Mix

Day 6:

Breakfast: Citrus Smoothie
Lunch: Salmon Salad Niçoise
Dinner: Spaghetti With Chickpeas Meatballs
Snacks/Desserts: Yogurt Parfait

Day 7:

Breakfast: Chickpea Scramble Bowl
Lunch: Egg Fried Rice
Dinner: Lentil Bolognese
Snacks/Desserts: Hummus

Day 8:

Breakfast: Banana-Coconut Smoothie
Lunch: Spinach And Eggs Salad
Dinner: Shrimp And Asparagus Salad
Snacks/Desserts: Roasted Chickpeas

Day 9:

Breakfast: Mocha-Banana Smoothie
Lunch: Sardines with Artichokes and Greens
Dinner: Veggie Burger with Avocado
Snacks/Desserts: Potato Chips

Day 10:

Breakfast: Sweet Peach Smoothie
Lunch: Asian-Inspired Peanut Noodles
Dinner: Broccoli and Cheddar Soup
Snacks/Desserts: Carrot Cupcakes

Day 11:

Breakfast: Spinach Omelet
Lunch: Coconut Veggie Wraps
Dinner: Bok Choy and Chicken Stir-Fry
Snacks/Desserts: Simple Banana Cookies

Day 12:

Breakfast: Belgian Waffles
Lunch: One-Pan Halibut
Dinner: Black Bean Stuffed Sweet Potatoes
Snacks/Desserts: Roasted Walnuts

Day 13:
Breakfast: Almond Quinoa
Lunch: Lentil Rice Soup
Dinner: Mushroom and Spinach Lasagna
Snacks/Desserts: Dark Chocolate Bites

Day 14:
Breakfast: Scrambled Tofu
Lunch: Turkey with Barley and Squash
Dinner: Tuna Vegetable Wrap
Snacks/Desserts: Baked Carrot Chips

Day 15:
Breakfast: Mixed Berry Smoothie
Lunch: Salmon Salad Niçoise
Dinner: Spaghetti With Chickpeas Meatballs
Snacks/Desserts: Yogurt Parfait

Day 16:
Breakfast: Citrus Smoothie
Lunch: Egg Fried Rice
Dinner: Lentil Bolognese
Snacks/Desserts: Hummus

Day 17:

Breakfast: Chickpea Scramble Bowl
Lunch: Spinach And Eggs Salad
Dinner: Shrimp And Asparagus Salad
Snacks/Desserts: Roasted Chickpeas

Day 18:

Breakfast: Mocha-Banana Smoothie
Lunch: Sardines with Artichokes and Greens
Dinner: Veggie Burger with Avocado
Snacks/Desserts: Potato Chips

Day 19:

Breakfast: Sweet Peach Smoothie
Lunch: Asian-Inspired Peanut Noodles
Dinner: Broccoli and Cheddar Soup
Snacks/Desserts: Carrot Cupcakes

Day 20:

Breakfast: Spinach Omelet
Lunch: Coconut Veggie Wraps
Dinner: Bok Choy and Chicken Stir-Fry
Snacks/Desserts: Simple Banana Cookies

Day 21:
Breakfast: Belgian Waffles
Lunch: One-Pan Halibut
Dinner: Black Bean Stuffed Sweet Potatoes
Snacks/Desserts: Roasted Walnuts

Feel free to adjust portion sizes based on your dietary needs, and remember to stay hydrated throughout the day!

Conclusion

You flipped the last page, fingers sticky with Balsamic-Glazed Roasted Cauliflower (that recipe alone is worth the price of admission). Your mind's humming, not just from the sugar rush, but from the possibilities. You can almost taste the sharpness, the clarity, the spark that the MIND diet ignited.

But here's the thing, this book isn't just a collection of recipes. It's a blueprint for a bolder, brighter you. You're not just cooking, you're building a fortress against fuzziness, a shield against forgetfulness. You're reclaiming your sharp edges, your wit, your zest.

Remember Aunt Jane, belting out show tunes in the supermarket? That's the music within you waiting to be unmuted. This book is the conductor, orchestrating a symphony of vibrant dishes that tickle your taste buds and nourish your neurons.

And the beauty? This isn't punishment, it's liberation. You're ditching the bland cardboard of "diet food" for feasts that celebrate your life. You're saying no to memory aids and yes to remembering where you left your keys (and the names of everyone at your next family reunion).

So, close your eyes. Imagine yourself a year from now. Sharper, bolder, a force to be reckoned with. That's not a fantasy, it's the future simmering right now on your stovetop. Now go on, open the fridge, grab that head of kale, and get cooking. Remember, the revolution starts on your plate. And believe me, the mind you build will be delicious.

Weekly Meal Journal

week OF: _______________

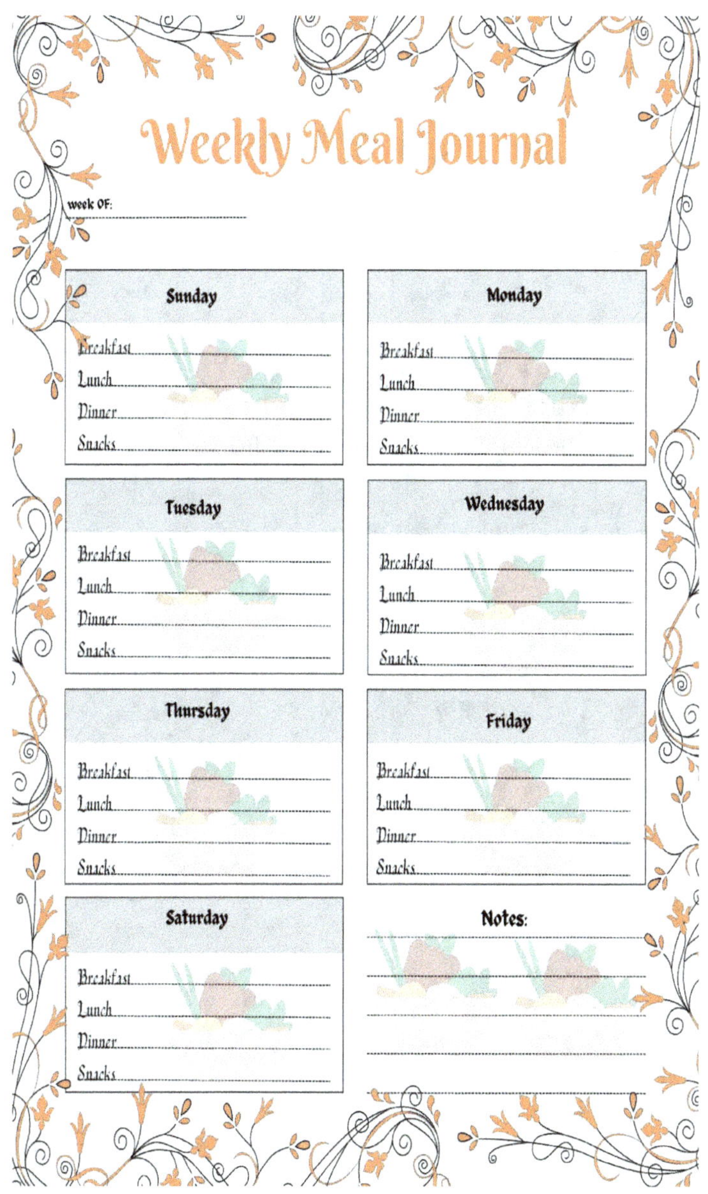

Sunday	**Monday**
Breakfast	Breakfast
Lunch	Lunch
Dinner	Dinner
Snacks	Snacks
Tuesday	**Wednesday**
Breakfast	Breakfast
Lunch	Lunch
Dinner	Dinner
Snacks	Snacks
Thursday	**Friday**
Breakfast	Breakfast
Lunch	Lunch
Dinner	Dinner
Snacks	Snacks
Saturday	**Notes:**
Breakfast	
Lunch	
Dinner	
Snacks	

Weekly Meal Journal

week OF: _______________

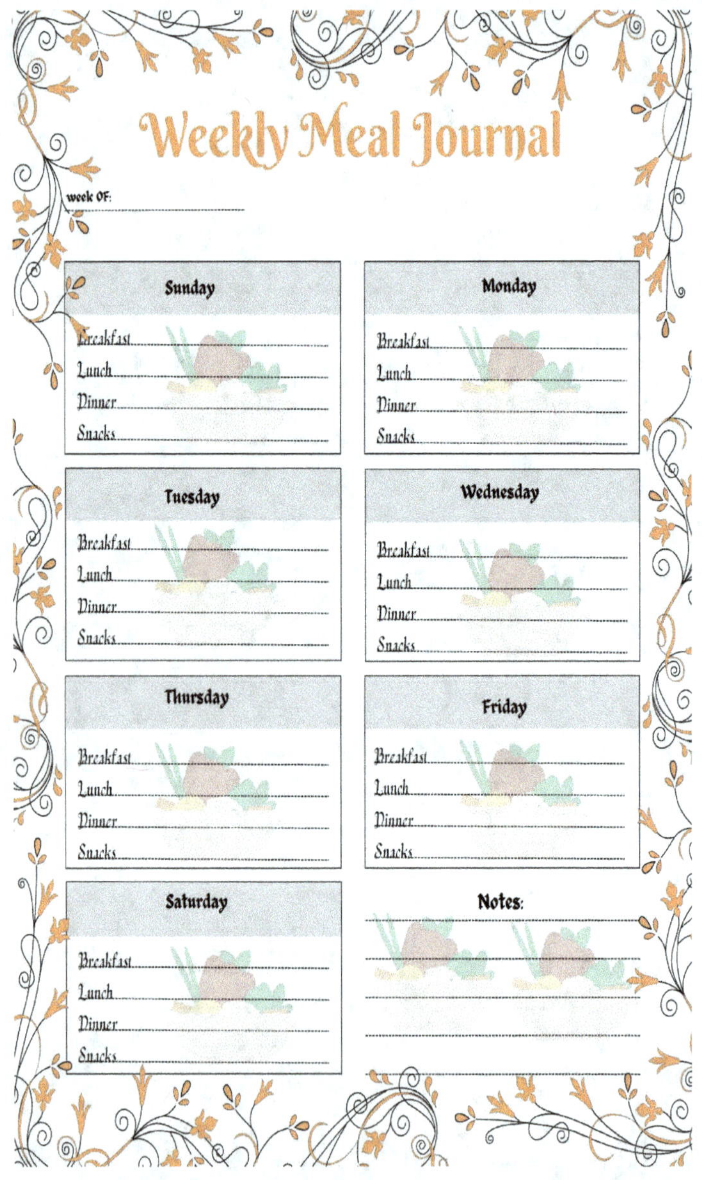

Sunday

Breakfast
Lunch
Dinner
Snacks

Monday

Breakfast
Lunch
Dinner
Snacks

Tuesday

Breakfast
Lunch
Dinner
Snacks

Wednesday

Breakfast
Lunch
Dinner
Snacks

Thursday

Breakfast
Lunch
Dinner
Snacks

Friday

Breakfast
Lunch
Dinner
Snacks

Saturday

Breakfast
Lunch
Dinner
Snacks

Notes:

Weekly Meal Journal

week OF: _______________________

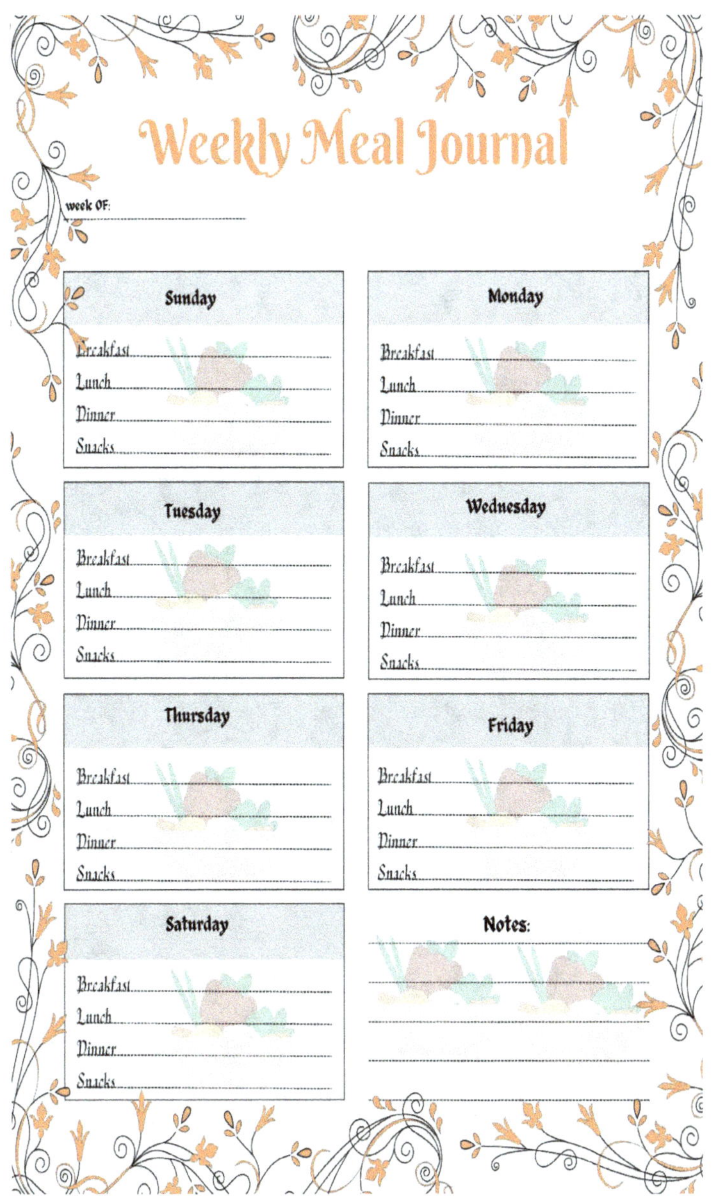

Weekly Meal Journal

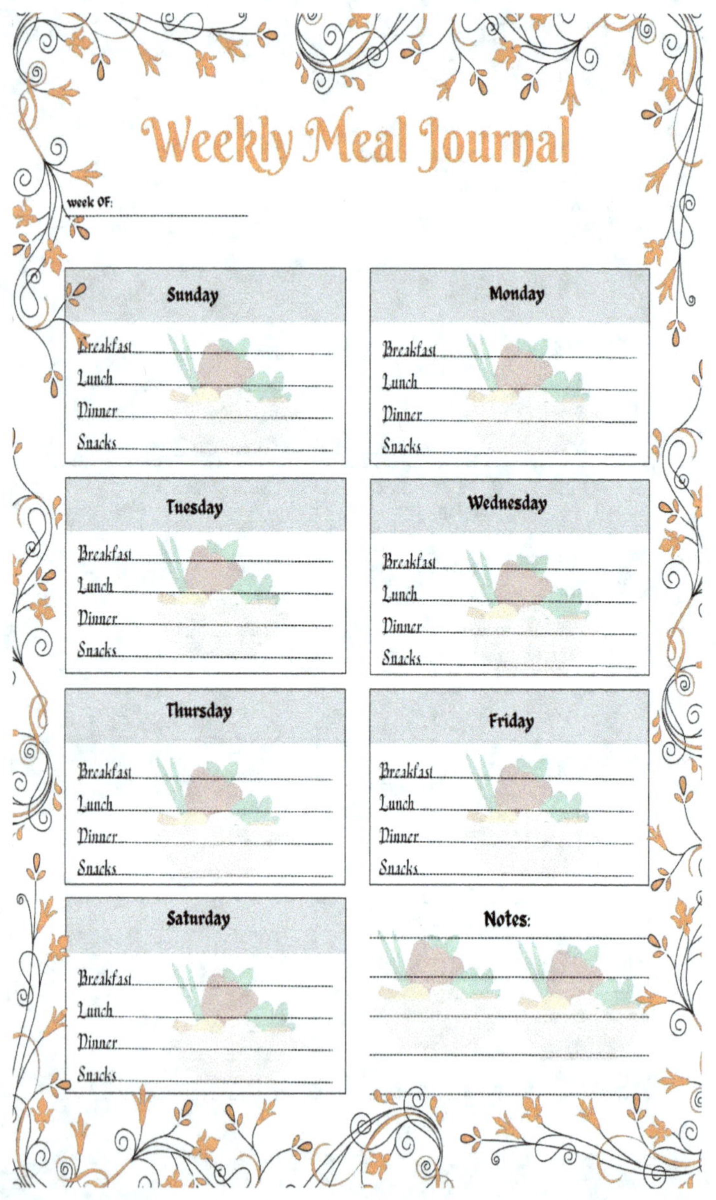

week OF: _______________________

Sunday
Breakfast ....
Lunch ....
Dinner ....
Snacks ....

Monday
Breakfast ....
Lunch ....
Dinner ....
Snacks ....

Tuesday
Breakfast ....
Lunch ....
Dinner ....
Snacks ....

Wednesday
Breakfast ....
Lunch ....
Dinner ....
Snacks ....

Thursday
Breakfast ....
Lunch ....
Dinner ....
Snacks ....

Friday
Breakfast ....
Lunch ....
Dinner ....
Snacks ....

Saturday
Breakfast ....
Lunch ....
Dinner ....
Snacks ....

Notes:

Weekly Meal Journal

week OF: _______________

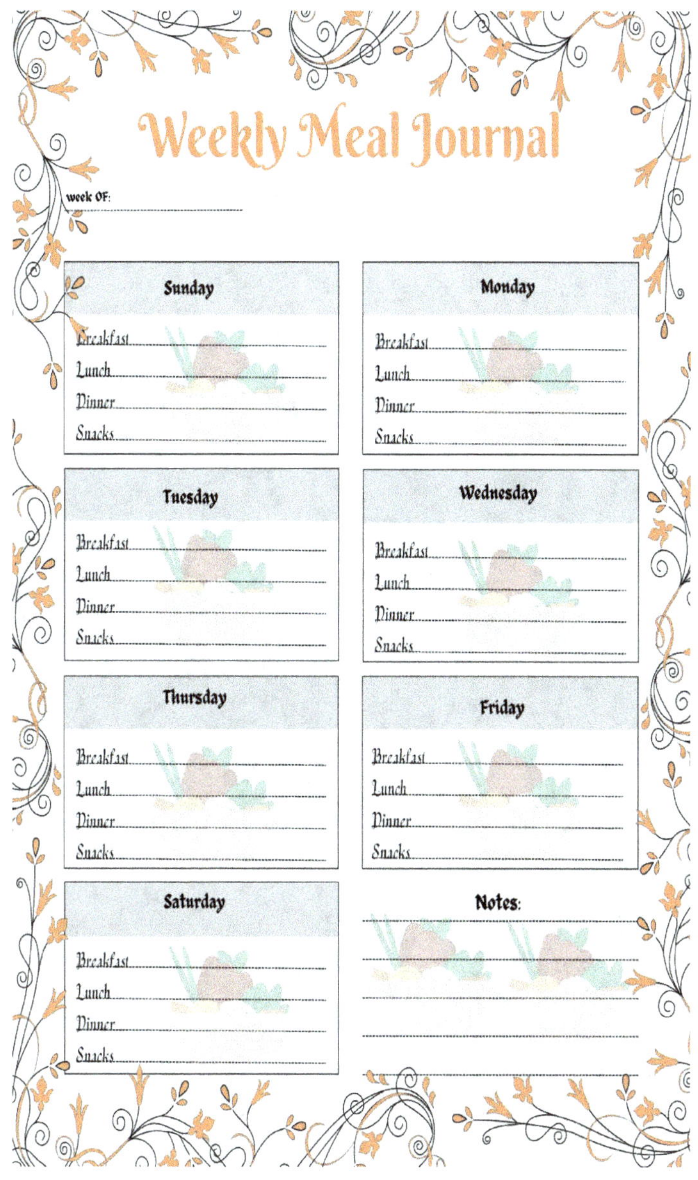

Sunday

Breakfast _______________
Lunch _______________
Dinner _______________
Snacks _______________

Monday

Breakfast _______________
Lunch _______________
Dinner _______________
Snacks _______________

Tuesday

Breakfast _______________
Lunch _______________
Dinner _______________
Snacks _______________

Wednesday

Breakfast _______________
Lunch _______________
Dinner _______________
Snacks _______________

Thursday

Breakfast _______________
Lunch _______________
Dinner _______________
Snacks _______________

Friday

Breakfast _______________
Lunch _______________
Dinner _______________
Snacks _______________

Saturday

Breakfast _______________
Lunch _______________
Dinner _______________
Snacks _______________

Notes:

____
____
____
____

Weekly Meal Journal

week OF: _______________

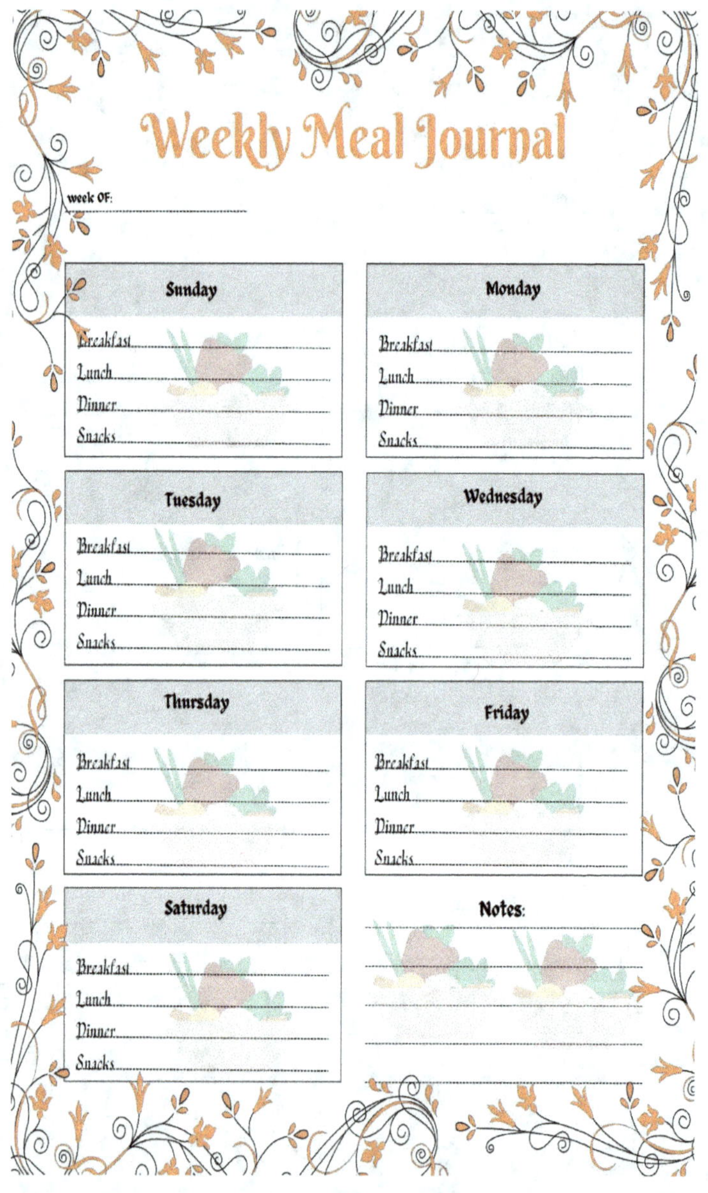

Sunday

Breakfast ....
Lunch ....
Dinner ....
Snacks ....

Monday

Breakfast ....
Lunch ....
Dinner ....
Snacks ....

Tuesday

Breakfast ....
Lunch ....
Dinner ....
Snacks ....

Wednesday

Breakfast ....
Lunch ....
Dinner ....
Snacks ....

Thursday

Breakfast ....
Lunch ....
Dinner ....
Snacks ....

Friday

Breakfast ....
Lunch ....
Dinner ....
Snacks ....

Saturday

Breakfast ....
Lunch ....
Dinner ....
Snacks ....

Notes:

Weekly Meal Journal

week OF: _______________

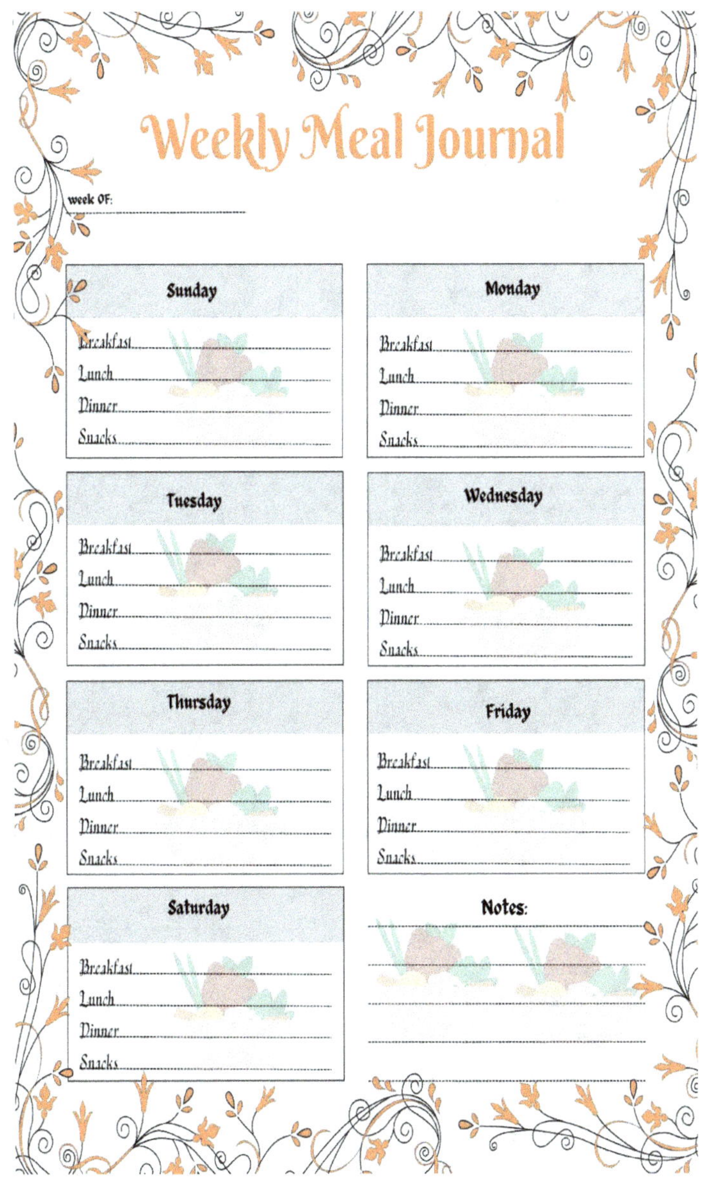

	Sunday		**Monday**
Breakfast		Breakfast	
Lunch		Lunch	
Dinner		Dinner	
Snacks		Snacks	

	Tuesday		**Wednesday**
Breakfast		Breakfast	
Lunch		Lunch	
Dinner		Dinner	
Snacks		Snacks	

	Thursday		**Friday**
Breakfast		Breakfast	
Lunch		Lunch	
Dinner		Dinner	
Snacks		Snacks	

Saturday

Breakfast
Lunch
Dinner
Snacks

Notes:

Weekly Meal Journal

week OF: _______________

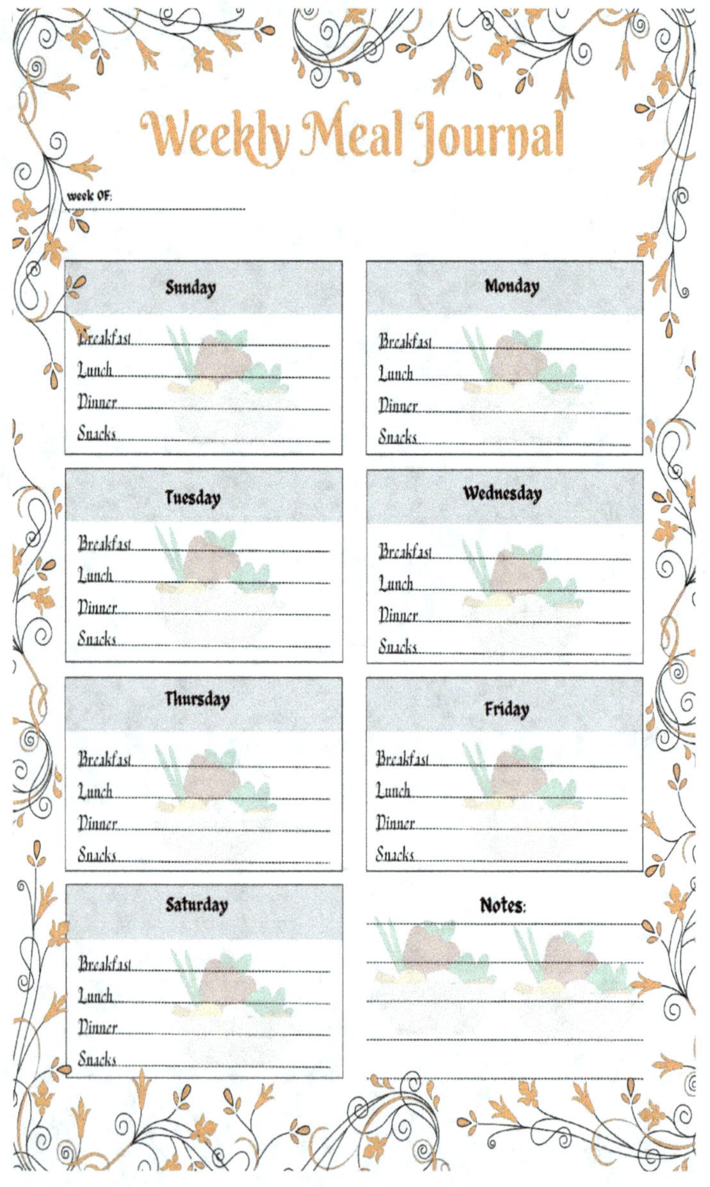

Weekly Meal Journal

week OF: _______________

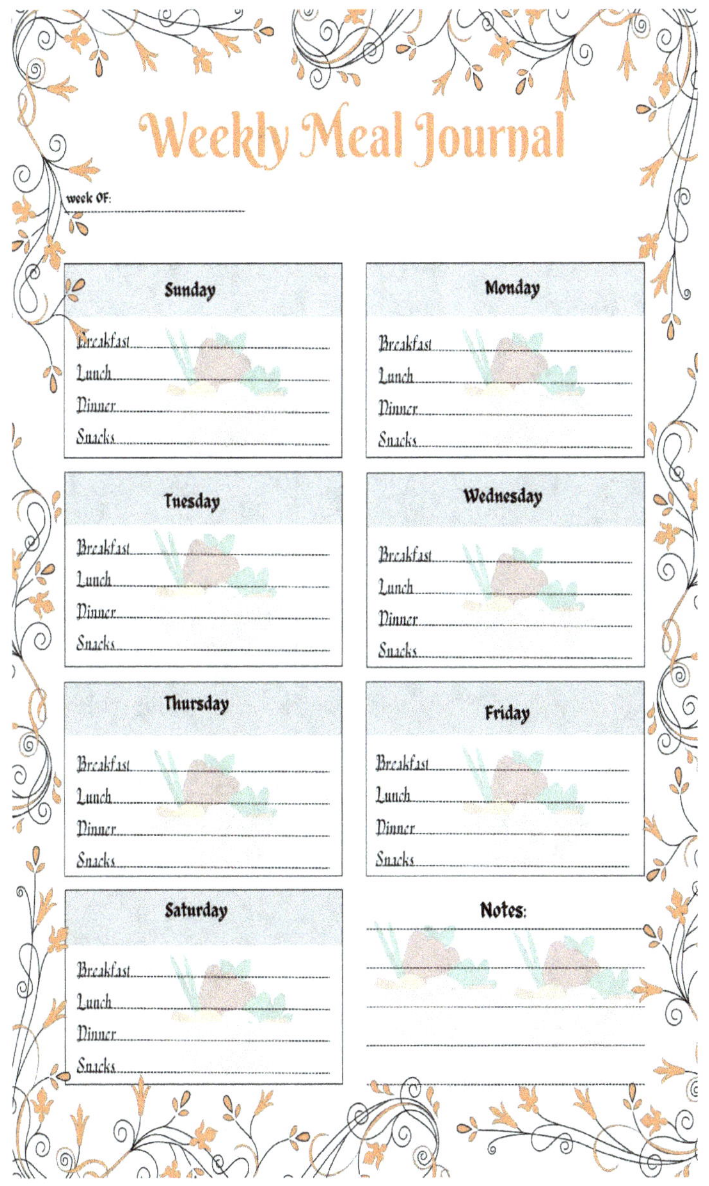

Sunday

Breakfast ....
Lunch ....
Dinner ....
Snacks ....

Monday

Breakfast ....
Lunch ....
Dinner ....
Snacks ....

Tuesday

Breakfast ....
Lunch ....
Dinner ....
Snacks ....

Wednesday

Breakfast ....
Lunch ....
Dinner ....
Snacks ....

Thursday

Breakfast ....
Lunch ....
Dinner ....
Snacks ....

Friday

Breakfast ....
Lunch ....
Dinner ....
Snacks ....

Saturday

Breakfast ....
Lunch ....
Dinner ....
Snacks ....

Notes:

Weekly Meal Journal

week OF: _______________________

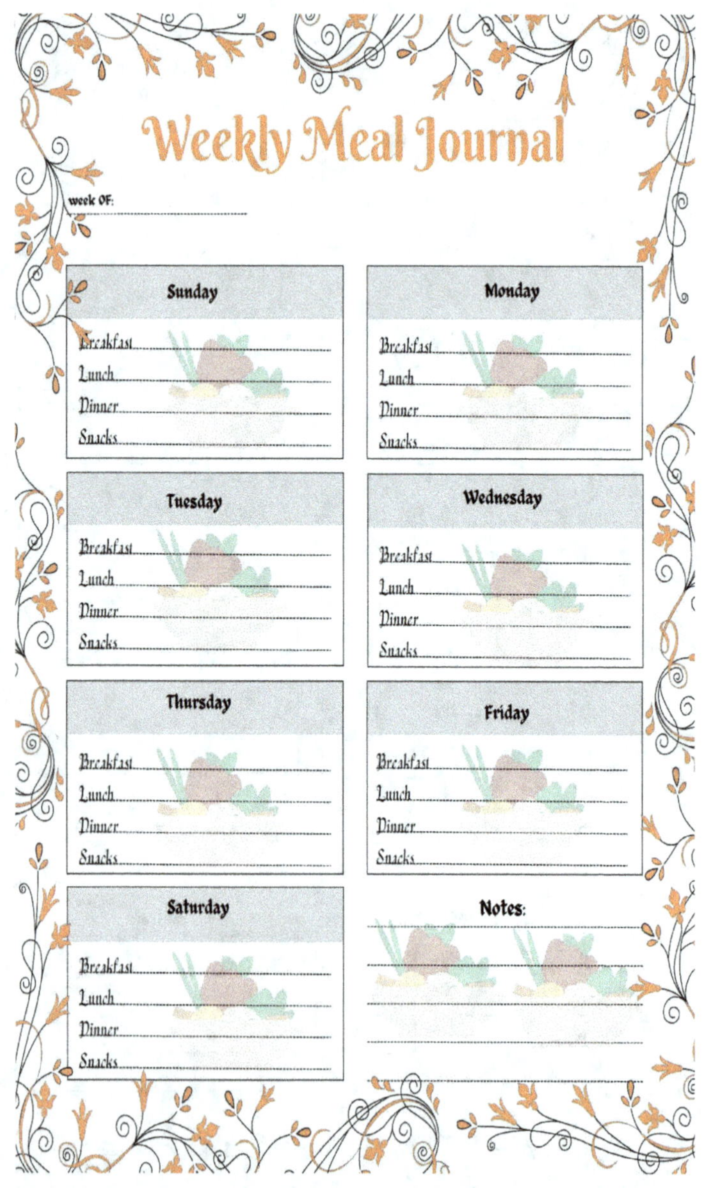

Sunday

Breakfast ....
Lunch ....
Dinner ....
Snacks ....

Monday

Breakfast ....
Lunch ....
Dinner ....
Snacks ....

Tuesday

Breakfast ....
Lunch ....
Dinner ....
Snacks ....

Wednesday

Breakfast ....
Lunch ....
Dinner ....
Snacks ....

Thursday

Breakfast ....
Lunch ....
Dinner ....
Snacks ....

Friday

Breakfast ....
Lunch ....
Dinner ....
Snacks ....

Saturday

Breakfast ....
Lunch ....
Dinner ....
Snacks ....

Notes:

Weekly Meal Journal

week OF: _______________________

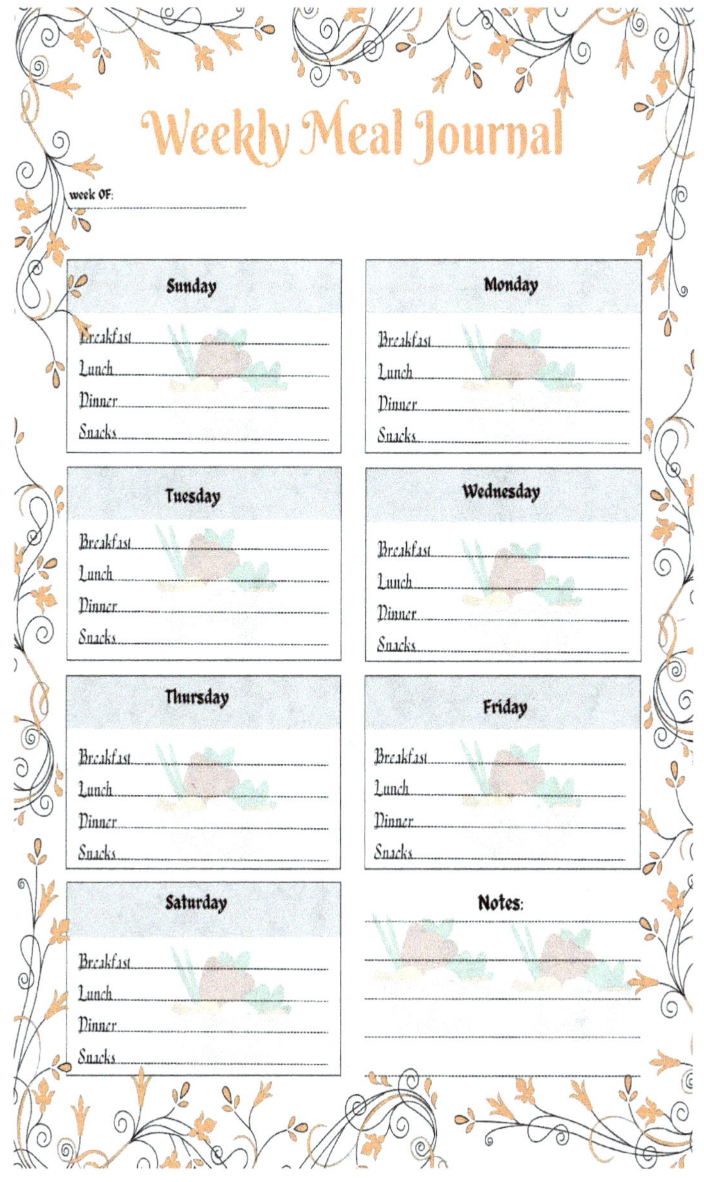

Sunday	**Monday**
Breakfast	Breakfast
Lunch	Lunch
Dinner	Dinner
Snacks	Snacks
Tuesday	**Wednesday**
Breakfast	Breakfast
Lunch	Lunch
Dinner	Dinner
Snacks	Snacks
Thursday	**Friday**
Breakfast	Breakfast
Lunch	Lunch
Dinner	Dinner
Snacks	Snacks
Saturday	**Notes:**
Breakfast	
Lunch	
Dinner	
Snacks	

Weekly Meal Journal

week OF: _______________

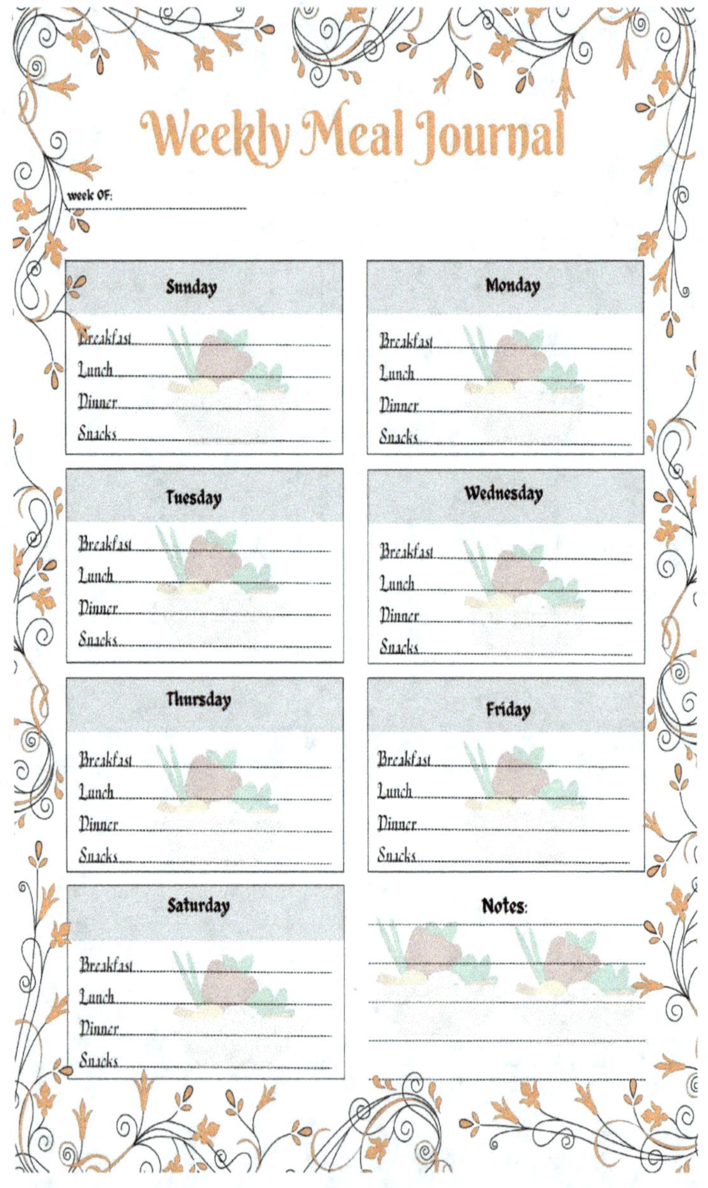

Sunday

Breakfast ....
Lunch ....
Dinner ....
Snacks ....

Monday

Breakfast ....
Lunch ....
Dinner ....
Snacks ....

Tuesday

Breakfast ....
Lunch ....
Dinner ....
Snacks ....

Wednesday

Breakfast ....
Lunch ....
Dinner ....
Snacks ....

Thursday

Breakfast ....
Lunch ....
Dinner ....
Snacks ....

Friday

Breakfast ....
Lunch ....
Dinner ....
Snacks ....

Saturday

Breakfast ....
Lunch ....
Dinner ....
Snacks ....

Notes:

Weekly Meal Journal

week OF: _______________

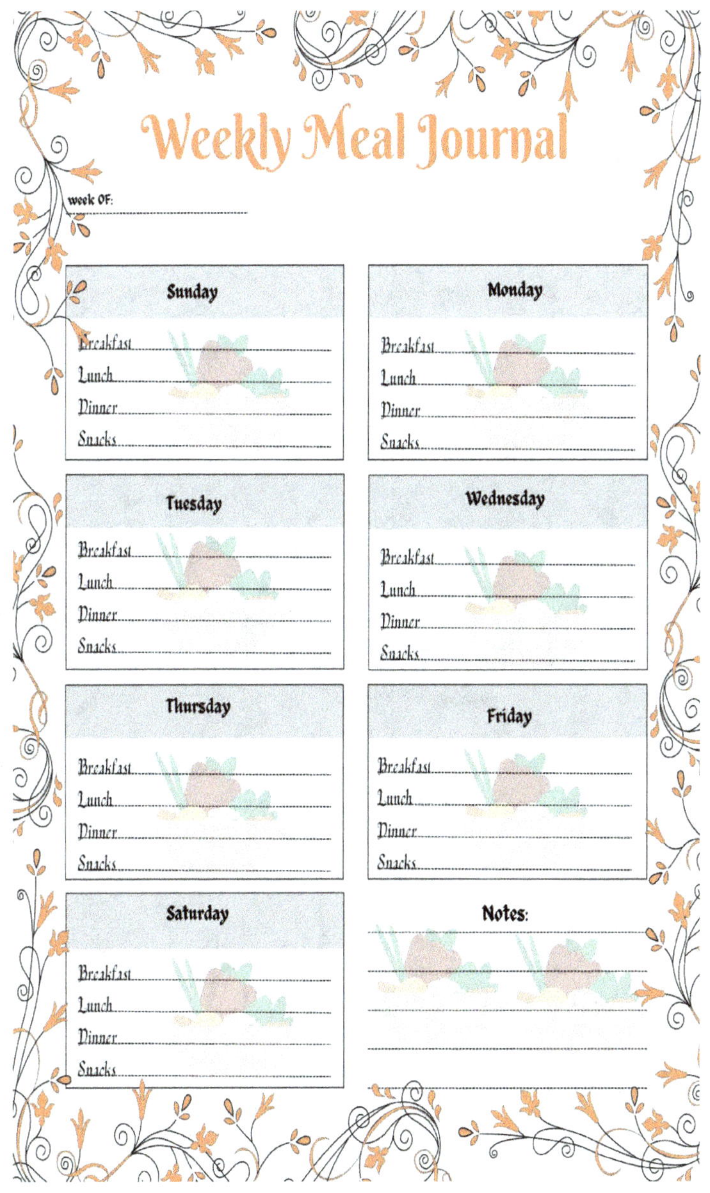

Weekly Meal Journal

week OF: ___________________

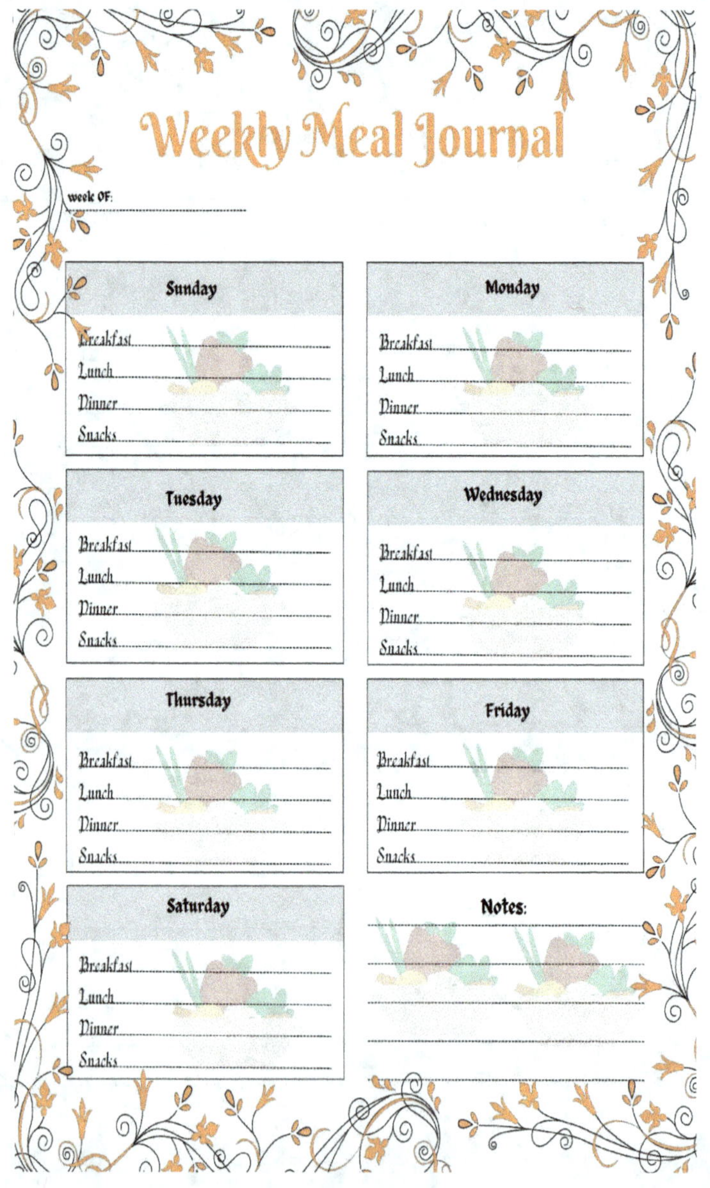

Sunday	**Monday**
Breakfast	Breakfast
Lunch	Lunch
Dinner	Dinner
Snacks	Snacks
Tuesday	**Wednesday**
Breakfast	Breakfast
Lunch	Lunch
Dinner	Dinner
Snacks	Snacks
Thursday	**Friday**
Breakfast	Breakfast
Lunch	Lunch
Dinner	Dinner
Snacks	Snacks
Saturday	**Notes:**
Breakfast	
Lunch	
Dinner	
Snacks	

Weekly Meal Journal

week OF: _______________

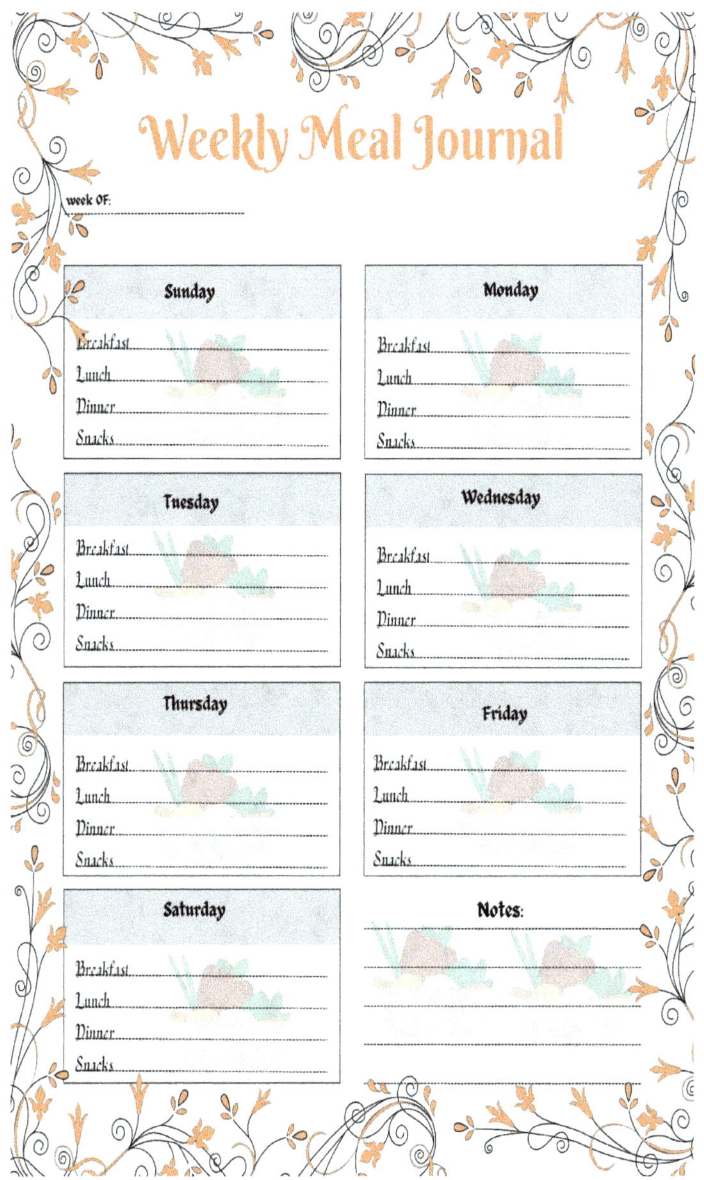

Sunday

Breakfast ....
Lunch ....
Dinner ....
Snacks ....

Monday

Breakfast ....
Lunch ....
Dinner ....
Snacks ....

Tuesday

Breakfast ....
Lunch ....
Dinner ....
Snacks ....

Wednesday

Breakfast ....
Lunch ....
Dinner ....
Snacks ....

Thursday

Breakfast ....
Lunch ....
Dinner ....
Snacks ....

Friday

Breakfast ....
Lunch ....
Dinner ....
Snacks ....

Saturday

Breakfast ....
Lunch ....
Dinner ....
Snacks ....

Notes:

Weekly Meal Journal

week OF: _______________

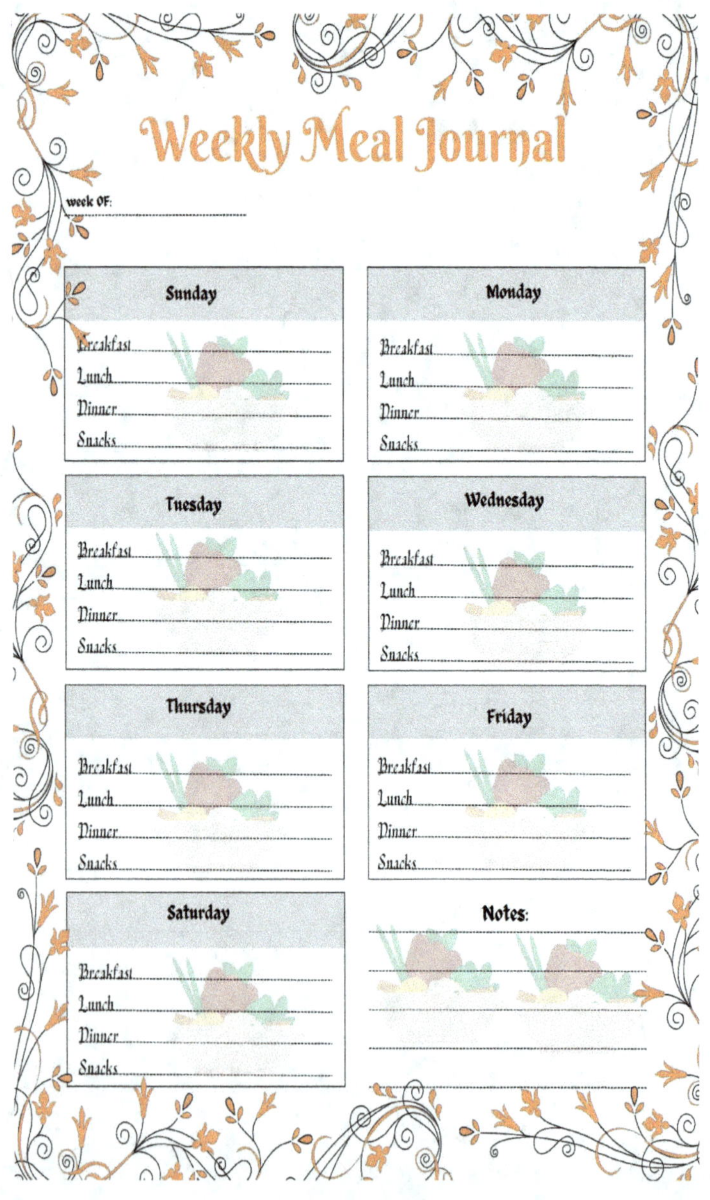

Sunday

Breakfast ______________
Lunch ______________
Dinner ______________
Snacks ______________

Monday

Breakfast ______________
Lunch ______________
Dinner ______________
Snacks ______________

Tuesday

Breakfast ______________
Lunch ______________
Dinner ______________
Snacks ______________

Wednesday

Breakfast ______________
Lunch ______________
Dinner ______________
Snacks ______________

Thursday

Breakfast ______________
Lunch ______________
Dinner ______________
Snacks ______________

Friday

Breakfast ______________
Lunch ______________
Dinner ______________
Snacks ______________

Saturday

Breakfast ______________
Lunch ______________
Dinner ______________
Snacks ______________

Notes:

____
____
____
____

Weekly Meal Journal

week OF: ________________

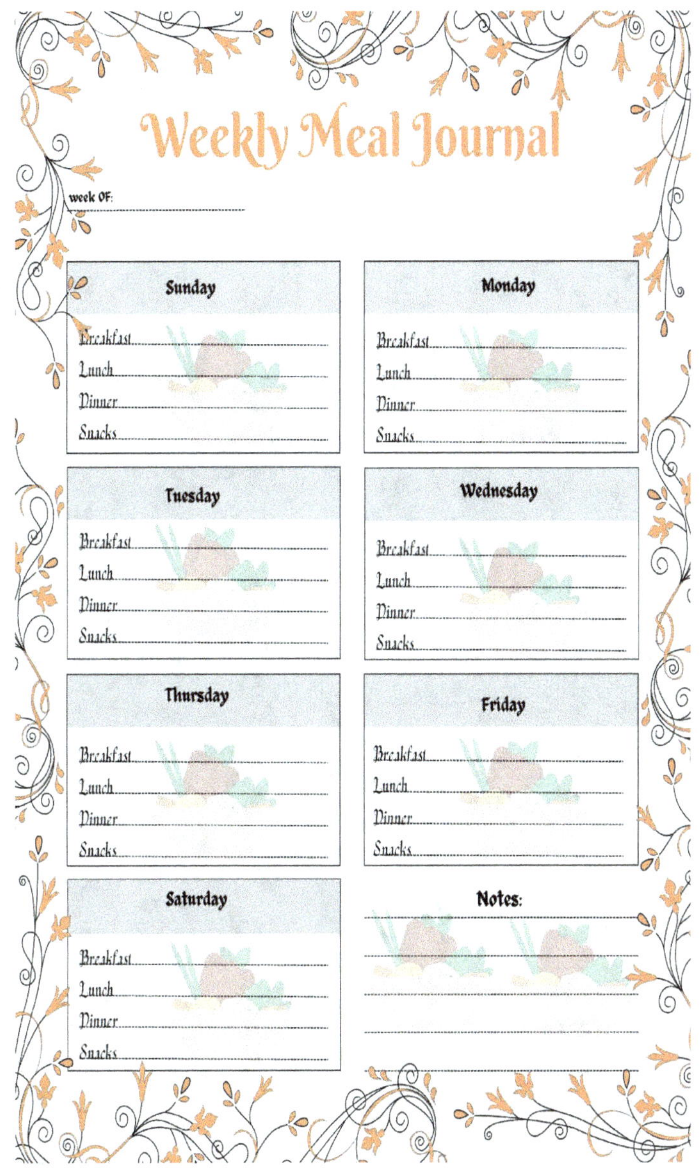

	Sunday
Breakfast	
Lunch	
Dinner	
Snacks	

	Monday
Breakfast	
Lunch	
Dinner	
Snacks	

	Tuesday
Breakfast	
Lunch	
Dinner	
Snacks	

	Wednesday
Breakfast	
Lunch	
Dinner	
Snacks	

	Thursday
Breakfast	
Lunch	
Dinner	
Snacks	

	Friday
Breakfast	
Lunch	
Dinner	
Snacks	

	Saturday
Breakfast	
Lunch	
Dinner	
Snacks	

Notes:

Weekly Meal Journal

week OF: _______________

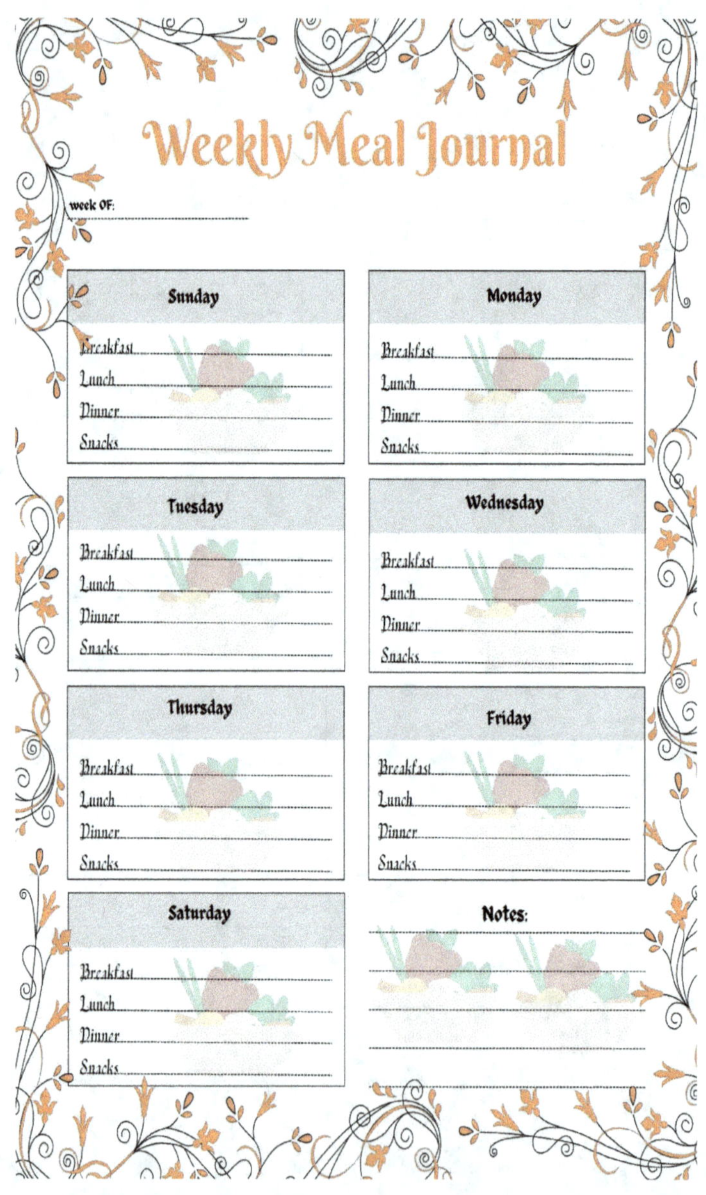

Sunday

Breakfast ....
Lunch ....
Dinner ....
Snacks ....

Monday

Breakfast ....
Lunch ....
Dinner ....
Snacks ....

Tuesday

Breakfast ....
Lunch ....
Dinner ....
Snacks ....

Wednesday

Breakfast ....
Lunch ....
Dinner ....
Snacks ....

Thursday

Breakfast ....
Lunch ....
Dinner ....
Snacks ....

Friday

Breakfast ....
Lunch ....
Dinner ....
Snacks ....

Saturday

Breakfast ....
Lunch ....
Dinner ....
Snacks ....

Notes:

....
....
....
....

Weekly Meal Journal

week OF: _______________

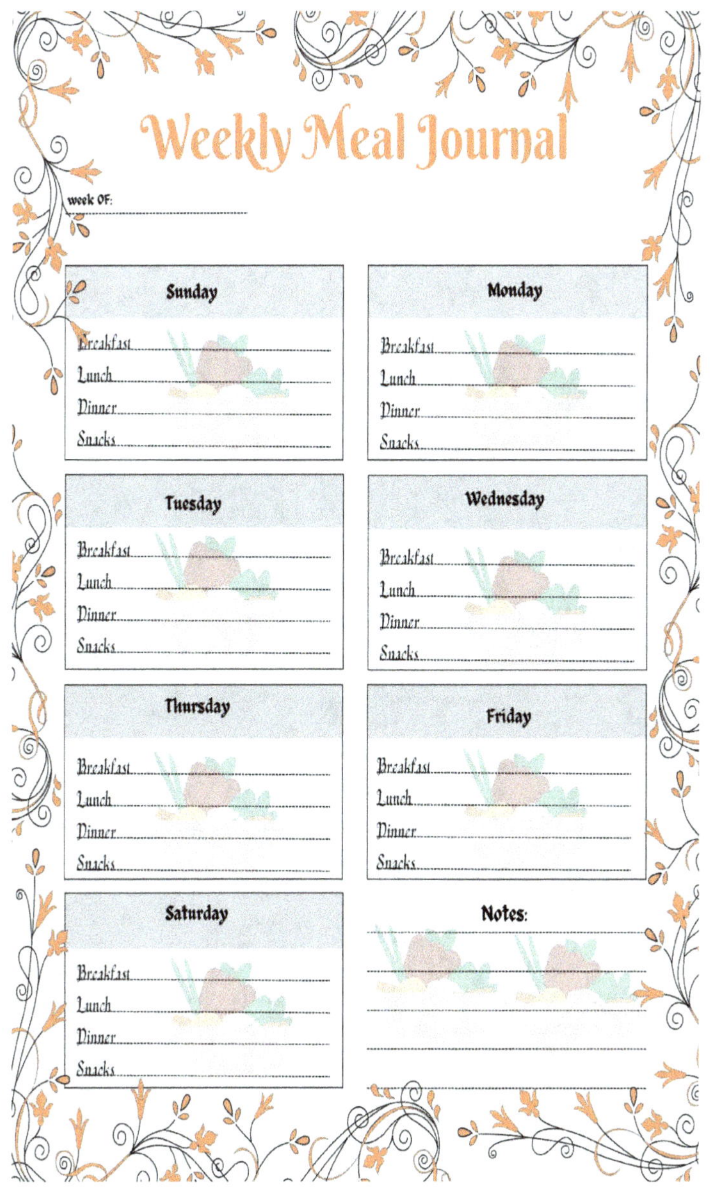

Sunday

Breakfast ....
Lunch ....
Dinner ....
Snacks ....

Monday

Breakfast ....
Lunch ....
Dinner ....
Snacks ....

Tuesday

Breakfast ....
Lunch ....
Dinner ....
Snacks ....

Wednesday

Breakfast ....
Lunch ....
Dinner ....
Snacks ....

Thursday

Breakfast ....
Lunch ....
Dinner ....
Snacks ....

Friday

Breakfast ....
Lunch ....
Dinner ....
Snacks ....

Saturday

Breakfast ....
Lunch ....
Dinner ....
Snacks ....

Notes:

Weekly Meal Journal

week OF: _______________

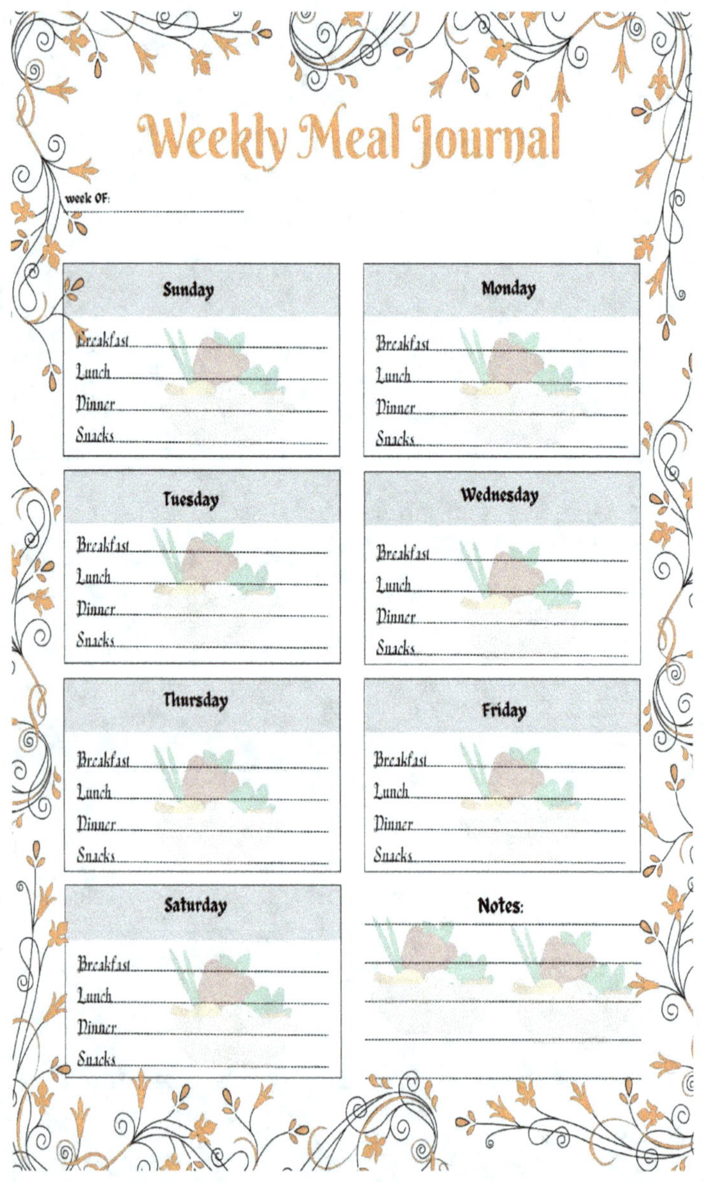

	Sunday
Breakfast	
Lunch	
Dinner	
Snacks	

	Monday
Breakfast	
Lunch	
Dinner	
Snacks	

	Tuesday
Breakfast	
Lunch	
Dinner	
Snacks	

	Wednesday
Breakfast	
Lunch	
Dinner	
Snacks	

	Thursday
Breakfast	
Lunch	
Dinner	
Snacks	

	Friday
Breakfast	
Lunch	
Dinner	
Snacks	

	Saturday
Breakfast	
Lunch	
Dinner	
Snacks	

Notes:

Weekly Meal Journal

week OF: ______________________

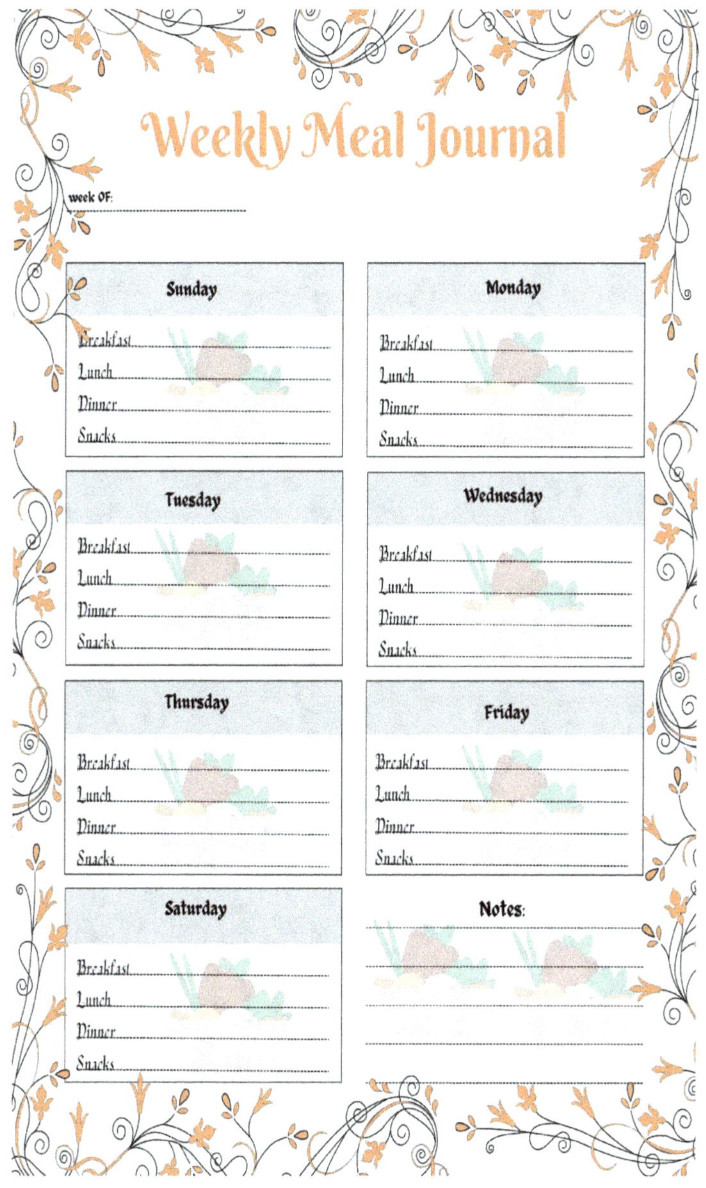

Sunday

Breakfast ....
Lunch ....
Dinner ....
Snacks ....

Monday

Breakfast ....
Lunch ....
Dinner ....
Snacks ....

Tuesday

Breakfast ....
Lunch ....
Dinner ....
Snacks ....

Wednesday

Breakfast ....
Lunch ....
Dinner ....
Snacks ....

Thursday

Breakfast ....
Lunch ....
Dinner ....
Snacks ....

Friday

Breakfast ....
Lunch ....
Dinner ....
Snacks ....

Saturday

Breakfast ....
Lunch ....
Dinner ....
Snacks ....

Notes: